The Other Side of Paediatrics

New Approaches to Care

We are beginning to realise that there is another side to patient care—the side which recognises the importance of patients as individuals and their social, psychological and emotional needs. These needs are frequently overshadowed by today's technically advanced, yet often impersonal, care.

The *New Approaches to Care Series* examines the other side of care in a practical and realistic way, recognising both the importance of such care, and the constraints which exist in hospital and in the community.

This approach aims to help nurses and other health professionals, both in training and in practice, to achieve more complete care of their patients.

Series Editors

June Jolly
Jill Macleod Clark
Will Bridge

THE OTHER SIDE OF PAEDIATRICS

A Guide to the Everyday Care of Sick Children

June Jolly, SRN, RSCN

Illustrated by Gillian Simmonds, ARCA

First edition 1981
Reprinted with corrections 1982

Published by
THE MACMILLAN PRESS LTD
London and Basingstoke
Companies and representatives
throughout the world

Typeset by Cambrian Typesetters,
Farnborough, Hampshire
Printed in Hong Kong

ISBN 0 333 29448 3 (hard cover)
     0 333 29449 1 (paper cover)

To sick children everywhere and
to all who have made this book
possible: patients, families and colleagues

Contents

Foreword

June Jolly is a nurse, a children's nurse, who has seen a great deal and felt a great deal. After many years of watching the hospital scene she has attained that rare thing, a capacity for understanding what is going on in a child of any age, what he is thinking or feeling and what he needs. She began by studying social sciences and then became a Child Care Officer. She spent twelve years in this arduous and often heart-breaking work. Her insights into family life drew her more and more towards the child himself and then to that special corner of childhood — illness and the hospital.

One of her earliest appointments was that of Night Sister at St. Christopher's Hospice. She has therefore experienced the nursing of people at the end of life, some of whom are about to leave it, as well as those at life's beginning. She has been a children's ward sister at St. Thomas's Hospital, London and the Brook General Hospital. In these posts with her great experience and knowledge of social work and family problems she was able to teach a new approach. A 'child', whether baby, toddler or of school age, is one part of a coherent whole — the family.

The long tradition (before Platt and even since) of viewing the child and handling him just as a very demanding little adult, had to be modified. It has, of course, always been the endeavour of paediatricians to inculcate in all hospital personnel a respect for the child's individuality, but June Jolly shows that it is only through taking him together with his family that this individuality can properly be seen.

Everything in this book is a record of the direct observation and experience of the author. What a refreshing story it is! Sweeping out old hide-bound ways of looking at things and obsessional adherence to traditional practices, and illustrating every point from her marvellous collection of examples. The first requisite of any treatment, she reminds us, is that it shall do no harm. We know we do harm, or at any rate cause suffering additional to the illness. We, the doctors and nurses, justify our rigid attitudes by pointing to the many dangers of the passage of a child through a hospital — anaesthesia, potent drugs and exactitude of dosage, cross-infection, accidents, exposure of children to sights that would be better concealed from them, and so on. But one does not find in this account of the handling of the sick child that any of these dangers are forgotten or that strictness for safety is disparaged; only that we can be understanding, liberal, relaxed and tolerant, and still be safe.

The book is written primarily for nurses (though by heavens the doctors and surgeons need it too!) and with the principal hope that it will help them to acquire, before during or after training, a *new attitude*.

Nurses experience early in their training that in giving their skill to adult patients, by their unselfish work, they evoke gratitude and affection in return. Children have no notions of gratitude (till they are much older), but nurses often sense the warm response of the child to whom they have given some specially understanding care. It is one of the unasked-for rewards of devoted people. But the new attitude is one which takes into account a much broader concept of the child to whom she will give this understanding care.

A child is dependent on his parents whether they are present or absent, and the very young child is utterly dependent. The nurse who can give her concern not just to the particular stress or need of the moment, but, as it were, beyond the child to all his 'appendages' — his parents (absent or present), brothers, sisters, school teacher, cat, possessions; his world in fact — she has the new attitude.

Family centred care is June Jolly's name for it.

Dermod MacCarthy, MD, FRCP, DCH
Formerly Consultant Paediatrician,
Stoke Mandeville, Amersham and High Wycombe
Hospitals, Bucks, and Honorary Paediatrician to the
Institute of Child Psychology, London.

Preface

What is the other side of paediatrics? For years it has been the accepted practice to nurse children in isolation from their families, their friends and their environment. Physical treatment has been excellent and staff have lavished much tender loving care on their patients. Every year medical and technical advances have made medical prognoses even better. But something vital has been missing. It is only in the last twenty years or so that attention has begun to focus on the child's other needs: for him to have his family, and more particularly his parents, with him at all times; room and freedom to play; access to education and facilities to meet his developmental requirements. Providing for these in a hospital setting required changes of approach, attitudes and expectations of staff and patients. Administrators too need to be involved in planning and providing a different kind of facility for children. It is this that I have called 'the other side of paediatrics'. It is so essential that one could well call it 'the human side'.

This book is written primarily for my fellow nurses as they have the 24-hour care of the children. It is their attitude that will determine how much families are really included in the care of their sick children. They create the atmosphere — whether welcoming and warm or clinical and cold. With skill and inclination to communicate at a child's level, a nurse can add enormous support to young patients and, in doing so, greatly increase her own job satisfaction.

Throughout the following chapters I have endeavoured to share my experiences over the years as I have struggled to respond to the sick children I nursed, who always wanted more than just to have their bodies mended, their diseases cured and their handicaps eased. It is my hope that it will be an encouragement to see that it is possible, gloriously possible, to meet these needs within an ordinary paediatric ward. If it also stimulates new ideas and innovations, and nursing staff to be more ambitious and courageous in over-coming obstacles, it will have been worth all the effort. It is because of this that I have tried to concentrate on practical issues including many of the everyday problems that may be encountered. I have also tried to suggest practical solutions, drawing on the experience both of colleagues and in a few instances describing specific projects designed to meet particular problems.

In 1974 I was privileged to receive a Florence Nightingale and Rayne Foundation Scholarship, which enabled me to visit many centres throughout Canada and the United States — North American experience is referred to in a number of chapters. References to the centres visited are recorded at the close of the chapter concerned.

This book is divided into three parts: 'New Approaches to Sick Children', 'Meeting the Needs of the Whole Child' and 'The Ward Team'. Although one might have expected to start with the needs of the child, it seemed important first to set the scene in which the new approach to sick children has been made, and then to establish the main concept of that change — family-centred care (Chapters 1 to 3).

In order to understand the needs of the child, a basic knowledge of child development is essential. For example, the process through which children under three years' old relate to adults is very complex. They are unable to relate to any adult except as a 'mother', and when a succession of adults take on the caring role the child attempts to develop such a relationship only to be passed on to another. Thus the anguish of losing the mother can be repeated many times over. If more nurses and doctors were aware of this problem there would be more support for ensuring that whenever possible young patients were not separated from their mothers even for short spells of hospitalisation.

One chapter is devoted to play because of the importance children attach to it, and specific 'hospital' play is discussed, as well as the types of play most acceptable to children with certain conditions. As communication with children of various ages is somewhat specialised, this is also discussed in a separate chapter. The need for the right environment and how to create it is the topic of Chapter 7.

Finally, Chapters 8 to 10 are devoted to the ward team — its functioning and organisation from the staff point of view. Students may not be prepared for the differences in paediatrics, for example, and the challenges this may bring. Moreover, the ward team may include a number of specialists of various disciplines and approaches to children. Their different functions are identified in the hope that their expertise will be better utilised and their place on the ward team ensured. These specialists may include the nursery nurse, the play specialist, the school teacher, the liaison health visitor, social worker, physiotherapist, occupational and speech therapists, dieticians, and district or community nurses. These 'specialists' join with the nurses and doctors, auxiliaries, receptionists, orderlies, ward hostesses and housekeepers to create the ward team. In some areas the teams may be augmented by a ward granny, family receptionist and members of the psychological services. A formidable team indeed, and when one realises that a number of different doctors, nurses and auxiliaries may be involved in nursing an individual child, it is not surprising that the child and his parents can be somewhat bewildered by the vast array of new faces they meet whilst in hospital.

For this reason it is vital that attempts are made to limit the number of people involved in the care of any individual patient. Case assignment, but preferably *family* assignment, can mitigate some of the fragmentation of care. When all approaches to the child can be made through the mother, she effectively buffers the onslaught and can protect her offspring from much of the fear that is so often its accompaniment. This is particularly relevant in the light of one recent study (Hawthorn, 1974) which showed that in only one week's stay in hospital, children received care from as many as 17 nurses, while in the best unit observed it was never less than 10.

There are considerable numbers of children who are still nursed in adult wards because of adult-orientated surgeons and a few physicians prefer to have all their patients in one place. This may save a few steps for the busy specialists – but at serious costs for their young patients. While children continue to be nursed alongside adult patients it will be extremely difficult and expensive to provide adequately for their special needs. Not only is it impracticable to provide the facilities necessary for many small groups of patients, but also the staff in these specialised units often remain unaware of the young patient's needs. Even if it is possible to include parents in some of the care, and provide living-in accommodation within the ward, it will be virtually impossible to change the timetable to suit a youngster, let alone to provide space for play, education and for maintaining good contacts with his peers and community events. The cost to the young patients is obvious. Children who are transferred from an adult area to a children's ward usually make better progress once they are in a place where they feel they 'belong'. The need for nursing children in paediatric wards is vital.

It has been my experience that this sort of enlightened care can be established and practised within the restraints and confines of general district hospitals, that the special needs of children do not have to be sacrificed to the needs of the majority, and that old buildings can be adapted, in some cases perhaps more easily than new ones. It is not a question of vast additional expenditure — in some areas, no new costs will be incurred, and in some there may even be savings. The main requirement is determination and perseverance by the nurses and other staff involved, backed by a sound basic knowledge of child developmental needs and enough imagination to see how best to use the resources available.

In most hospitals there are many improvements in child-nursing practice still to be made, often major improvements but awaiting only the vision and action of the staff involved. It is because of this that I share my experiences in the following pages. Nursing sick children is the most rewarding and satisfying job I know. Heartache, frustration, hard work there will be, but it can be such fun.

Hove, 1980   J.D.J.

Acknowledgements*

This really isn't 'my' book at all. Without the help and encouragement of my friends and family it probably would never have reached the printing press. Without my sister Gill's sensitive illustrations it might not have been understood. Her sharing not only in the message the book contains, but also in its communcation, will, I hope, engender further ideas and innovations, in ways which will continue to improve care for the sick child.

It is therefore my joy to give honour where honour is due. To Jill Macleod Clark, whose enthusiasm first inspired and who then cajoled and generally bullied me into writing this book; to Margaret Atkin who burnt the midnight oil with me and gave me courage to go on when I really felt it was impossible; to Richard my brother and his wife Alison whose support and encouragement was there to fall back on at every turn; to my good friend and colleague Edna Anderson whose experience in the care of children and their families is now much greater than mine — I would like to give sincere thanks.

I am privileged to have had the professional advice and counsel of many notable people: James and Joyce Robertson who have given so graciously of time and expertise and who taught me much of my understanding of young children, especially those vulnerable 'under-threes'; Peg Belson, founder member of NAWCH† – the National Association for the Welfare of Children in Hospital — with whom I have shared concerns for so long and to whom I owe more than I can say; Susan Harvey, who gave me many insights from her unique knowledge of play for sick children and lent me such

---

* *Purely for the convenience of readers the pronoun 'he' has been used to describe children of either sex. For the same reason all staff are referred to in the female gender.*

† *The National Association for the Welfare of Children in Hospital, Exton House, 7 Exton St., London, SE1.*

valuable assistance over the years. My thanks are due too to
Sally Huband, whose concern for paediatric nurses and their
training I admire and who gave me much pertinent and
practical advice. I cannot omit mentioning my dear friend
Vivian who out of love, painstakingly deciphered all those
scribbles and typed the whole manuscript so well, and Julie
Robson who so patiently typed and retyped the final copy.

Lastly I want to pay tribute to Dr Dermod MacCarthy
who has borne the brunt of revising the text, making
suggestions from his wealth of experience with characteristic
sensitivity, humility and meticulous care. It was he who first
had the courage to include families in the contemporary care
of sick children. To me it is the greatest honour that he
should consent to write a foreword.

Part One:

New Approaches to Sick Children

1 Why a New Approach to Caring for Sick Children is Necessary

'It's like this. When I was a child I
spoke and thought and reasoned as a child
does. but when I became a man my thoughts
grew far beyond those of childhood and now
I have put away childish things.'

The Living Bible

Introduction

Children really are different. It is indefensible to regard them
as miniature adults. It will require positive effort on our part
to get on to their wavelength, to understand their thinking
and the way they reason.

The challenge of paediatric nursing today is in meeting
the needs of the whole child. This means not only attending
to his physical care, but also paying attention to his thoughts,
his feelings, and his need for his family. It has to be recognised that children think differently from adults. Their
reasoning may appear illogical and their understanding is
limited and grows only with experience. One of the tasks of
anyone caring for children is to provide a climate in which
growth can continue, even under adverse circumstances such
as a hospital stay. Bearing in mind that over a quarter of the
child population of Britain spends at least one night in
hospital before they reach the age of seven, these issues are
crucial. If we fail, if we get it wrong, we may not get another
chance. The sensitive caring for the 'other side of paediatrics'
the needs of the whole child, body, mind and spirit, cannot
be overstressed.

Historical Background

It is only comparatively recently, within the last hundred years in most countries, that children have been admitted to hospital at all. Until then hospital care was limited to 'useful members of society'. It was felt anyway that the child's prime need was to be with his mother. The death-rate was high. A century ago children under ten accounted for over 40 per cent of the deaths in London alone. Gradually, special children's hospitals were founded, and understanding of the disease process of childhood increased. Alongside this advance came the awareness of the dangers of cross-infection. Although initially parents were included in the care, as life expectancy for even sickly youngsters improved, the physical care of children took priority. On the grounds that visitors brought infection, parents were later excluded except under very restricted conditions. Often they were merely allowed

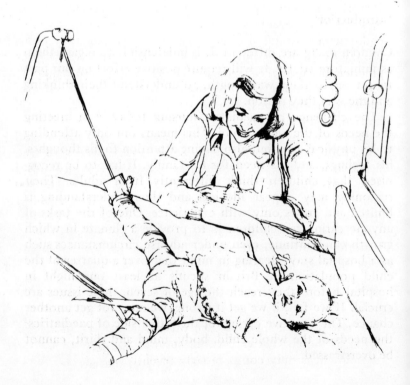

to look through the window and then only after the children were asleep. Visiting might be weekly, or even once a month. This unfortunate situation gradually changed, especially after the risks of infection were found to be more within the hospital than from outside.

However, it is only since the 1950s that researchers such as Bowlby (1953), Freud (1952) and Robertson (1952), recognised and demonstrated the widespread and damaging emotional effects which separation can have on young children. Parents too over the years have reported how disturbed their children have been after even short spells in hospital. Evidence of this may be short-lived, such as nightmares, or 'not letting the mother out of sight'. Others report that their child has not been the same since, for various reasons. This, of course, may not be entirely due to separation or lack of mothering, but neither can it be totally dismissed.

Partly as a result of their findings, the now famous Platt Report was published in 1959 and unequivocally recommended that parents should have unlimited access to their children in hospital. Even in maternity and isolation units, visiting is now established as a regular and advantageous practice because it is seen that patients get better quicker given the stimulus of welcome visitors. However, in spite of the recommendations, access to children even today is still limited in various ways.

When visiting is restricted it is said it is because it will disturb the patient and there are still many hospital staff who feel that exclusion of parents is justified on these grounds. I have never found it so. Parents in my experience are only too eager to do anything that will benefit their child, providing they are told how, and are quite able to assist, say, in keeping a post-operative tonsillectomy patient quiet and peaceful — something that the staff are not always able to do especially if he is crying for his 'Mum'.

The Needs of the Child

Whereas it has long been accepted that the physical well-being of the child is vital to his survival and performance as an adult, it is only comparatively recently that attention has been given to the emotional and psychological aspects of his care.

THE NEED FOR CONTACT WITH PARENTS

Awareness of the sick child's emotional dependence on his mother has become better understood as a result of the films of James and Joyce Robertson. *A Two-Year Old Goes to Hospital* (1952) highlighted the severe but typical psychological deterioration in a hospitalised child and the increasing disturbance in her relationship to the mother. This film showed dramatically how she turned away from her mother and how the child found it difficult to re-establish trust and express pent-up anxiety. Although she was seen as a 'good' child this film exploded the myth that the good child is contented.

This was followed in 1956 by a second film *Going into Hospital with Mother*, a practical demonstration of the positive difference it made if mothers could stay with their children in hospital. It also depicted the importance of staff attitudes; this was shown clearly by the ward sister's taking the mother into the kitchen and encouraging her to use the facilities as 'she would at home'. The second film was made at a small hospital where the far-sighted paediatric staff had put into practice the lessons learnt from the first disturbing film.

Gradually over the intervening years and encouraged by the publication of the Platt Report (1959) more and more hospitals have been opening their doors and allowing freer access to their children. Most now offer some form of overnight accommodation but still not enough for all parents of pre-school children to be admitted. The fact that even where free access is provided it is not always used is usually more a reflection of the attitudes of staff who still fail to realise the enormous importance of family support for the children, than reluctance or inability of parents to use the facilities offered.

The Robertsons have in recent years publicised the needs of those children who, for one reason or another, cannot have their parents with them. In typical dramatic visual form they have contrasted the experiences of the unaccompanied child with that of a child for whom a substitute mother has been found to stand in for the absent parent. The security provided for a vulnerable child by such a 'substitute mother', a devoted caretaker, can make a dramatic difference. In response to this challenge attempts are now being made to provide such care throughout the western world, with a variety of experimental schemes already in operation. For example, foster grandparents are used for this purpose in some American states; ward grannies are being recruited in New Zealand; the counsellors in Dutch hospitals are providing for this need too in a limited way. Some schemes at present being tried in Britain are described in detail on p. 11— 13 but there are few totally adequate schemes which really provide the round-the-clock care that a mother gives her sick child. However good a one-to-one relationship, it is doubtful that two or three hours a day will really satisfy the pre-school child, who needs to have someone all the time.

THE NEED FOR CONTACT WITH THE REST OF THE FAMILY

Children not only need the presence of parents, but the sense of belonging that comes with the special relationships they have with brothers and sisters. This is of increasing importance as the child develops. For all but infants, and possibly toddlers under two, brothers and sisters and any other older relatives who make up the nuclear family provide reassuring contact. Often brothers and sisters seem to have more rapport with a sick child than their parents. In some large families the elder brother or sister is the one already providing the mothering and they can then be an acceptable substitute to live in. Not only does the sick child need to see his brothers and sisters but the siblings themselves also need reassurance about the one in hospital. Incidentally, this can be educational should at a later stage they need hospital treatment.

DEVELOPMENTAL NEEDS

Children have very different needs at varying stages of their development. These are discussed further in Chapter 4. Whereas safety and security will always need to be considered as children become mobile, they require space for exploring, playing, learning, as well as letting off pent-up energy. As they are less articulate in voicing needs, empathy and skilled observation will be necessary in order to satisfy them. Communication must be geared to their powers of understanding and couched in terms they recognise. Help to express their feelings and experiences may be given by providing suitable play materials. It is only as we recognise that children's developmental needs are just as specific as their physical ones, that we will realise the tremendous importance such facilities are to them.

Meeting these Needs

Hospitals today offer a more sophisticated and comprehensive service than ever before. This is as true for paediatric patients as for any other section of the community. There is a growing tendency to integrate health care and for the emphasis to be put on preventative rather than curative medicine. 'Primary care' seeks to provide a service within the home, and hospital is seen as an episode in the care of the sick child. Nevertheless, children and their parents will probably always need to call on the hospital services in a crisis. It is at this point when they are most vulnerable that paediatric staff are naturally most involved. How can the services available best be utilised to meet the very special needs of the future generation? We cannot ignore the child's developmental needs, or his need for contact with his family as well as his parents.

Dr MacCarthy in a paper to the British Paediatric Association (1974) acknowledged that it is not possible for doctors to establish close and direct relationships simply on conventional ward rounds and he deplored the lack of one-to-one relationships achieved by most paediatricians with their young patients. This is equally true for most nurses who must expect to do more than purely clinical work if they are to establish adequate relationships with the children. In looking at potential ways in which to meet these important needs the starting point must be an acceptance by staff in all disciplines that a new approach is needed. This will involve for many, a change of attitude. Indeed, in my experience such changes in attitude are the real need and the usual stumbling-block — not shortage of cash or resources.

MAKING CARE MORE PERSONAL

Providing for the multitudinous needs of sick children calls for the expertise of many 'specialists' of various disciplines. This in itself works against the need of the young child to have a minimum number of people intimately involved in his care. Unfortunately specialists tend to be concerned only with a bit of the child and do not always feel they have time to be involved with the child as a person. Unhappily, not all specialists are conversant with the developmental needs of their young patients. Little training is given in these matters though this is beginning to improve.

One little boy of five put it succinctly when he reported after a hospital visit:

'They looked at my ears, they looked at my throat, they looked at my tummy, but they didn't look at me.'

André, aged eight, complained:

'My name is not "Hey you" my name is not "Little Boy", my name is ANDRÉ.'

In response to a recent survey on how children see their hospital experiences one ten year old summed it up for the group saying:

'There's no one to look after you. Everyone is too busy to listen to what you want.'

What he didn't say, but probably meant, is that he didn't feel there was anyone to listen to how he felt — let alone to alleviate his fears (*Which?* Report on Children in Hospital, 1980).

Individual care

The sheer number of nursing personnel in a hospital ward creates its own problems. As working hours are shortened, nurses change shifts more often. The idea of case assignment can never be truly implemented if only because of the shift system. The nursing process will help because of its accent on planned on-going care. But in most of the children's wards of this country it is difficult to limit nursing care and attention of any one child to a few nurses, let alone 'one's own nurse'.

In one hospital I visited in Canada the problem had been solved within the ward team. By changing over to 12-hour shifts, working similar hours in total, it meant that duties were spread over 3½ days, instead of the usual 5. Two nurses shadowing one another could then be responsible for the nursing care a child would need during his 'normal waking hours'. By careful allocation and team participation this voluntary scheme proved popular with the child and parents. The nurses found it gave them more job satisfaction and, although some said the hours at first had seemed long, they came to prefer it. The medical staff were enthusiastic even though it meant they could not approach their own patient without the special nurse in tow. But they had full reports and all their queries answered as she was always fully in touch. Some amazingly good results were observed. The recovery rate was quicker, despite the fact that this experiment took place on a neurosurgical ward. A number of patients were discharged who would not normally have been expected to be able to go home at all.

Yet this system of individualised nursing did not require an increase in the number of staff. The nurses selected children they felt likely to benefit from the scheme. It did not preclude the member of staff from helping with other duties or patients and she was able to carry her share of the workload. Such innovations could surely be extended?

INVOLVING THE FAMILY

One might have expected to discuss the involvement of families as the first priority in meeting the needs of the child in hospital. The reality is that, however much we might like every child's family to be involved, the need for nursing care remains. Nursing may be able to be done through the parents, but it is still the nurses' responsibility to provide that care, however it is achieved.

If family-centred care is to be practised certain adaptations both of the hospital facilities available and the management of the ward must be implemented. Parents who are 'living-in' or even visiting all day have different expectations and sometimes unrecognised needs. This is discussed in detail in the following two chapters.

Working alongside families will prove stressful on occasions and involving the parents will mean that a great deal of patience may be necessary to teach and inform the parents of how they can best help. By being sensitive to their point of view and anticipating some of their needs — for a rehydrating drink, or a quiet sit away from the busy ward, even somewhere to hang warm outdoor clothes, will quickly turn even diffident parents into allies as everyone works towards the recovery of the child patient.

SUBSTITUTES WHEN THE FAMILY IS NOT AVAILABLE

In 1973 James and Joyce Robertson speaking at the Annual Conference of NAWCH (the National Association for the Welfare of Children in Hospital) made a plea for *all* children under four admitted to hospital without their mothers to receive full-time substitute mothering, on the grounds that this can greatly diminish separation distress in young patients and would give them stable relationships and a haven of safety from the fears and frights of the hospital ward. When implementation of this was discussed there were reservations about providing 'foster parents' for unaccompanied children. It was decided to try to experiment with an older 'granny type' of volunteer surrogate mother.

The ward granny
It is sometimes possible to find a volunteer free to devote his or her time to doing what a good mother would do for her child in hospital — a 24-hour day job! Usually such a person is likely to be older and free from the stringencies either of

_mployment or family commitment, In one hospital in which I worked we had just such a 'person, a 'typical granny' figure — rosy-cheeked, bespectacled, round and motherly. She came originally in response to the need of a small road-traffic victim, whose mother and brother had been killed in a car

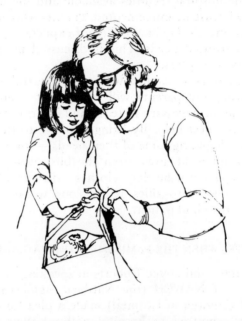

crash. She stayed by his bedside until he recovered consciousness and then, apart from short periods when his father was able to travel up for a visit, she cared for him until he recovered. Initially it was merely holding his hand, but it soon progressed to stories, helping to bath and coaxing him to eat. She remained to encourage and rejoice as he got back on his feet and regained his confidence.

Although it is tempting to share a 'granny' between two or three needy children, this just isn't good enough. One has only to be reminded of normal sibling rivalry to realise that unrelated children are certainly not going to be happy to share their 'gran' with anyone else. And in any case it defeats the object of the one-to-one relationship needful. In some hospitals the voluntary organiser can recruit such a person.

In others the wards have found their own — often a retired member of staff.

Experimental nursery nurse role

Interesting research has been conducted at a long-term orthopaedic hospital where concern was felt about the number of young toddlers and pre-school children. They were being nursed in the main ward which was a thoroughfare for many of the hospital personnel. Was the constant exposure to different people emotionally damaging? Nursery nurses were allocated to perform all the parenting tasks the young child would normally receive from his mother and involvement of other staff was drastically curtailed. The young patients were moved out of the busy part of the ward and attempts were made to recreate a quieter and more personal atmosphere reminiscent of a private home. The care of these children was restricted as much as possible, the nursery nurse being the one constant figure. Although it was not possible to give true continuity of care with existing staffing methods, even with this modified approach the report suggested that the children made more healthy normal progress. So much so that the experimental period has been indefinitely extended and is now ward policy for this age group.

Summary

If we are to implement the spirit of the new approaches to nursing sick children, each member of the ward team will need to be absolutely sure of the importance of the family to the individual child, in meeting his physical, emotional and developmental needs. Without a clear understanding of the child's basic needs at various stages it will be impossible to see beyond the obstacles and to overcome the problems that arise when they seem to conflict with the traditional facilities provided in hospital. Although this may apply more to those working in general district hospitals, we must still re-examine some of the time-honoured practices in the children's hospitals too.

We are still a long way from providing a comprehensive

child-orientated paediatric service, in which the family is able to function competently enough to meet the sick child's needs. We are a long way too from fully implementing the concept that all children under four require their mother all the time; that most children under five require their mother all the time; that some children of any age will also require their parents to stay with them. Is it just idealism to think that this is possible? Long-term goals for this were accepted as far back as the 1950s, but I believe that even today any paediatrician, any nurse, any administrator can effect changes that will allow these long-term goals to be realised.

Today's children may never have had it so good – but is it good enough? Unless we believe that these emotional and developmental needs are as vital to the child as his need for food or a bed, our answer must be 'No'. Unless we also act upon our convictions, our answer must still be 'No'.

References

Bergmann, T. and Freud, A. (1965). *Children in Hospital*, New York, International Universities Press.

Blake, F.G. (1954). *The Child, His Parents and the Nurse*, Philadelphia: Lippincott.

Bowlby, J. (1953). *Child Care and the Growth of Love*, Harmondsworth: Penguin.

Branstretter, E. (1969). 'The Young Child's Response to Hospitalisation, Separation or Lack of Mothering', *Am. Journal of Public Health*, 59, 92–97.

Committee on Child Health Services, (1976). *Fit for the Future* (The Court Report), London: HMSO.

Court, D. (ed.) (1970). *Paediatrics in the Seventies*, Nuffield Provincial Hospitals Trust, Oxford University Press.

Fagin, C. (1966). *The Effect of Maternal Attendance during Hospitalisation on Post-Hospital Behaviour*, Philadelphia: F. Davis.

Freud, A. (1952). 'The Role of Bodily Illness in the Mental Life of Children', *Psychoanalytic Study of the Child*, 7 August 1969.

Hawthorn, P. (1974). *Nurse I Want My Mummy,* London, Royal College of Nursing.

Hospital for Sick Children (Great Ormond Street) (1854). *How to Nurse Sick Children,* London: Longmans.

Jolly, J. (1974). 'The Ward Granny Scheme', *The Nursing Times,* 11 April 1974.

MacCarthy, D. (1962). 'Children in Hospital with Mothers', *The Lancet,* 24 March 1962, 603—608.

MacCarthy, D. (1965). 'A Parent's Voice', *The Lancet,* 18 December 1965, 1289—1291.

MacCarthy, D. (1979). *The Under Fives in Hospital,* National Association for the Welfare of Children in Hospital.

Mason, E.A. (1965). 'The Hospitalised Child. His Emotional Needs', *New England Journal of Medicine,* 272, 406—414.

Ministry of Health and Central Health Services Council (1959). *The Welfare of Children in Hospital* (The Platt Report), HMSO.

Ormeland, E. and J. (1973). *The Effects of Hospitalisation on Children,* Springfield, Illinois: Thanas.

Provence, S. and Lipton, R.C. (1962). *Infants in Institutions,* International Universities Press.

Prugh, D.G., Staub, *et al.* (1953). 'A Study of the Emotional Reactions of Children and Families to Hospitalisation', *American Journal of Orthopsychiatry.*

Robertson, J. (1952). *A Two-Year Old Goes to Hospital,* Ipswich: Concord Films (New York Film Library).

Robertson, J. and J. (1970). *Young Children in Brief Separation,* London: Tavistock Publications.

Robertson, J. and J. (1973). 'Substitute Mothering for the Unaccompanied Child', *The Nursing Times,* 29 November 1973.

Rutter, M. (1972). *Material Deprivation Re-Assessed,* Harmondsworth: Penguin.

Solnit, A.J. (1960). 'Hospitalisation. Aid to Physical and Psychological Health in Childhood', *American Journal of Diseases of Children,* 99, 155—163.

Stacey, M., Dearden, R., Pill, R. and Robinson, D. (1970). *Hospitals, Children and their Families* (Report of a Pilot Study), London: Routledge & Kegan Paul.

Which? Campaign Report (1980). Children in Hospital.
Wolff, S. (1969). *Children under Stress,* Harmondsworth: Allen Lane.

Places Mentioned

Brook General Hospital, Woolwich.
Children's Hospital, Montreal, Quebec, Canada. The Big Sister Programme on Neuro-surgical Unit.

National Orthopaedic Hospital, Stanmore, Middlesex.

2 Family-Centred Care

Introduction

By nature, all human beings start life within family units. Children instinctively call for 'Mummy' and 'Daddy' at the first sign of trouble or anxiety. In spite of these obvious truths, many otherwise excellent children's homes, hospitals or maternity units, have for years practised what amounts to 'parentectomies', the cutting-off of parental contact, in the name of progressive and therapeutic care. We have forsaken the 'doing what comes naturally' for the pursuit of objective clinical demands, albeit with the best of intentions. But what use are good intentions if we ignore the emotional repercussions of what we do or what we omit to do? In our 'scientific' concern we have neglected the equally important, if not vital, role of the family. TLC, the tender loving care that the nurse is taught to lavish on her patients has been treated as the right approach. So it is. It fails only insomuch as it is thought to be in any way an adequate substitute for the tangible presence of the child's mother and father.

The nurse today no longer has to act in place of the parents but has an enhanced and even more challenging role in working alongside the family whose child is ill. It needs to be recognised that no child can be treated really adequately in isolation from his family and home. In fact, when the family work with the medical and nursing staff towards the child's recovery, the experience for the child is better and return home may be sooner than is normally possible. Learning to do this poses many problems, particularly in a ward situation within the highly structured environment of an acute hospital. For the whole ward team — medical, nursing and para-medical — there are new concepts to assimilate, different skills to develop and, for many, attitudes will change as the accent on care becomes family-centred and veers away from being purely child-orientated.

Visitors or Non-Visitors

As parents and siblings are included in care, they lose their status and role as visitors. No longer can they be regarded as outsiders who are 'allowed' or even welcomed into the ward. While they remain visitors there is always the option to 'turn them out' when the going gets tough, the ward is busy, the doctors are doing a round, or even the cleaners are washing the floor. Sometimes the domestic staff actually request that parents do not visit until the wards have been cleaned; the doctors say they prefer to take blood tests and do their rounds before the parents come; nurses suggest parents are asked to leave because of bed-time, rest hour and so on. These arise because the role of the parents is imperfectly understood and indeed without such understanding they often sound very reasonable requests.

Adapting Hospital Services to Family Needs

In most hospitals there are arrangements for relatives of seriously ill patients to obtain a meal, rest or stay the night and administrators are usually pleased to be able to provide these. They are often less pleased, however, when these services are requested for the majority of children under five years, even those requiring admission for one or two days, as well as for the very ill. Totally adequate facilities are likely to be found only where it is appreciated that parents contribute to treatment, emotional well-being and recovery. Requests for regular meals, sleeping accommodation that is more than the temporary 'Put-U-Up', seldom attract enthusiastic support when resources are already overstrained. Even in new hospitals designed for flexible care the premium on rooms may mean doctors face the dilemma of allocating the 'seminar' room or office for parents' rooms at the expense of their own requirements. Nooks and crannies can more often be found in old buildings. I was fortunate to be able to convert a disused linenry into a kitchenette for the parents' use. But it is never easy; every inch of space may need to be fought for. Justification must be given to show that such use constitutes a higher priority than that of its competitors. So one needs to be fully convinced of the need before embarking on a campaign to improve facilities. The problems recede, however, when parents become accepted as part of hospital treatment. This is not to say that parents need to be given *carte blanche* to do what they like in disregard of the other needs of the ward, the myriad requirements of other patients and smooth housekeeping — but very few parents are like this.

What Parents Need

What sort of provisions do parents living in with their children really need? There are units up and down the country where the best is provided. There are other places where it is basic.

In a few long-stay hospitals serving huge catchment areas, purpose-built bungalows or caravans have been provided for visiting families. In some instances the patients join the family for the day or weekend. Special Care Baby Units are also beginning to provide accommodation in this way. One maternity hospital has had a flat for many years where patients can stay and 'get to know their baby' before final discharge; a 'half-way house' where the family can be as independent as they choose, but where professional help is instantly available via an internal telephone.

When considering family-centred care the needs of the other children must also be recognised. Some parents find themselves intolerably torn between the needs of the child in hospital and those of the siblings at home. This is frequently the case when there is a toddler and a breast-fed infant. It is not so impossible as it may sound to provide family rooms where the healthy sibling can be given board and lodging, allowing the parent to be with them both. Because no other care is provided the cost of this is minimal. In at least one hospital this has been in operation for 15 years or more. When there are spare beds in the ward these can be used too.

Parents are more concerned with the freedom to be really involved than in 'three star' hotel living. This is borne out by the fact that some of the best-appointed units are under used, whilst others are always finding there are more families wanting to stay than there is room. Although, when asked, many will say all they need is somewhere to lie down for a while and if possible somewhere to make a cup of tea, it is quickly discovered that life is made much easier for staff and families if reasonable facilities can be found.

SOMEWHERE TO SLEEP

A room where parents can 'let their hair down', express anxiety and grief out of sight of the children, or just have a rest, will relieve the rise of tension that often accompanies parents living in the same room as their child. Married couples need privacy at times, especially when they face the long ordeal of their child's surgery or disease. To provide parents with bedrooms as an alternative to sharing a cubicle with the sick child is much appreciated once the child has settled and is less acutely ill, so long as it is within calling distance and within the ward. Anything further away will heighten anxiety. When parents do have a room the staff find it easier too as they are not always under foot and their belongings do not clutter up already overcrowded areas.

SOMEWHERE TO EAT AND DRINK

A kitchenette or beverage point where snacks can be made will be much used. The freedom to make a cup of tea at any time of day or night will help parents to relax and feel more 'at home'. It is not uncommon for dads to come straight up to the hospital after work without stopping for a meal. If mums can make a quick snack in their own kitchenette this solves the problem. Many hospitals do not allow visiting parents to eat in the staff canteen, only resident ones — thus excluding Dad! Some mothers spend all day in the wards but because they go home to sleep and are 'not resident', they cannot get any refreshment unless there is a patients' shop or visitors' canteen. Even when these are available the opening hours are often limited and inconvenient for parents who have to fit in with the ward timetable.

SOMEWHERE TO BATH

Bathing and washing needs should be considered. It is seldom

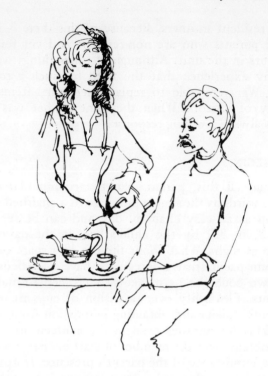

convenient for parents to use the children's bathroom. When newly delivered mothers are living-in and have only partially healed episiotomies there may be medical reasons for daily baths which will have to be disinfected before use. When parents stay in the unit for more than a few days, washing of smalls and even shampooing of hair may be requested. Where possible, a bathroom solely for parents' use should be allocated. It needs to be remembered that dads need to be made just as welcome as mums and often elect to 'do the night shift', so a shaving point will be most useful. Toilets may, of course, be requested by any visitor.

SOMEWHERE TO SIT

Units able to provide a sitting-room for parents sometimes find it needs to be kept locked to stop pilfering and keys are given to resident mothers. Because of this there is no place for those parents who are non-resident and yet remain for many hours in the unit. Although at times things were 'lost' it was my experience that the need for such a room was essential. We were able to replace necessary items by the generosity of visitors. When they knew what was wanted there was always a willing response.

HOW TO BEGIN

Having said all this, parents can be accommodated in the children's wards by the simple purchase of a chairbed that will double up as an easy chair by day and can be set up (see Chapter 3, p. 35) by the child's bed, in the dayroom, or playroom at night. What about the use of a spare bed in the ward? Some paediatric wards regularly have spare beds. Maybe one or two could be permanently sacrificed to make room for parents. Flexibility over provision of cups of tea, using the patients' toilets and obtaining permission for a person to get breakfast or another meal in the canteen are relatively minor problems once the member of staff in charge has understood the importance of the parent's presence. Hospitals may find, as more regular and substantial use is made of these facilities, that planning and procedural changes will be necessary. They may need time to adjust to these new attitudes, but one is on firm ground in Britain as there are numerous circulars from the Department of Health and Social Security (DHSS) which give support to these concepts (notably HM 71(22)).

Meeting Parent's Own Needs

As parents become part of the responsibility of the ward team their needs will become more apparent. Parents themselves need time and care, and some provision for their own support. For instance, telephones get more use in a children's unit than any other wards of the hospital, so I am told. Newly delivered mothers have definite physical needs and on occasions are bona fide patients in their own right (see chapter 3).

THE PROBLEM OF ENOUGH TO DO

Many parents feel totally redundant in the ward. They are always busy in their own homes with cooking, cleaning, mending and caring for the family. Many combine this with an outside job and have to organise their day precisely in order to keep the family going. If staff utilise this often un-tapped pool of voluntary labour, it can be to the benefit of all grades of staff, and not least to the parents themselves. The children, too, find it more normal to see Mum doing things and not sitting intently eyeing their every move, or becoming edgy with the unaccustomed strain of enforced idleness. Roy Meadows, in his study of resident mothers, describes his report as 'the captive mother', and quotes at least one who described her stay as 'like being in prison'. When her child is acutely ill, or being barrier nursed, she may have her hands full in assisting the nursing, or occupy-ing the isolated youngster. There may, however, be long periods of relative inactivity.

HELPING THE STAFF

Nursing staff may find themselves stretched to the limit to meet the nursing needs of the patients and find it difficult to make time even to direct the willing mother to what she can do to help. Mending cuddly toys, sewing on buttons and tapes, putting away the laundry, helping with the drinks or tidying the toy cupboards are jobs that usually do not cause any member of staff to feel their own job is being threatened, a point to remember in these days when unions are alert for potential threats to their members' jobs. Nurses on the other hand rarely have these concerns. On many occasions I have not only been grateful that there were parents to help, but aware that without their help it would have been a physical impossibility to provide even rudimentary care for the children on the ward. Once I had 34 children under two to administer medicine to and to feed with only two members of staff to help. That the children were all tucked up, warm, dry and fed was entirely due to some wonderful and co-operative parents. As far as the children were concerned, and I suspect the parents too, that particular evening was most satisfactory.

INDIVIDUAL DIFFERENCES

As families are invited to continue caring for their sick children in the wards, one is confronted with numerous family differences. These differences may be in standards of discipline, bathing, feeding, bedtime or even expectation of parents as regards their child's behaviour. Obviously there must be a common denominator for planning the patient's day and this is discussed more fully in Chapter 8. It can be a time to observe cultural differences and so enhance one's understanding. It can also be an unrivalled opportunity for teaching good practice and encouraging the young and unsure parents in the handling of their own children. Where families have specific problems it may be possible for one of the specialists in the ward team to help (see Chapter 3).

Tracey, a four-year-old child with syndactyly was admitted to the children's ward. Her mother was a highly strung woman, guilty about her child's condition which she later admitted she somehow felt responsible for. When she was with the child she made constant demands on her; smacking and trying to control her without success. Tracey screamed, disobeyed her mother and was a nuisance. As soon as her mother left she calmed down and became pleasant, playing with other children and happily complying with the group, cooperating with the nurses. The staff felt it would be better if the mother did not come in. On the surface, one would have to agree. Because I was sure in my own mind that the child and mother should be together, that when discharged they would have to be together anyway and this child was inevitably to be readmitted on at least two subsequent occasions for surgery, I felt we should persevere. Our aim would be to help the mother feel less threatened and to encourage her to relax.

The staff made a plan of action: the social worker's help was enlisted to help the mother sort out some of her own anxieties; the play specialist was asked to give special attention to Tracey's need to express herself. The mother was encouraged to participate in the activities in the playroom and also with the nurses. On subsequent admissions there was no recurrence of the problems or of the staff adverse reactions to Tracey or her mother's relationship. It seemed that our efforts had been effective.

STAFF INVOLVEMENT

It is a fairly new concept to nurse sick children in a hospital environment through and alongside parents. Young nurses and doctors coming into the paediatric unit may find this exposure to the 'critical eye' of a worried parent very threatening indeed. Learning to handle the unpredictable and sometimes uncooperative patient who cannot be reasoned with may be stressful enough. It can be magnified if it involves new techniques or intricate procedures such as finding a scalp vein or applying a urine collecting bag on a warm, moist and wriggling bottom. In our defensive attitude we think the parent is criticising our aptitude. In reality most young children object and cannot be expected to realise our ministrations are for their own good.

As parents are taken into the confidence of the staff and understand some of the technical difficulties such misunderstandings evaporate. Try explaining why it is necessary to hold the child's arm absolutely still and invite the parent to divert the child's attention whilst the test is being made. Take time to do so in a quiet and calm manner, otherwise the parent may catch the stress and not the sense of what you are saying and it will be hard for them to remain calm. No one can take the place of a calm confident parent, but one that is het-up and anxious can have the reverse effect. When the mother is too worried, too distressed, she is not equal to participating. The nurse will then have to spend time with both of them before she says 'I'll hold you for Mummy'. This will allow the mother to withdraw or the child can be taken to the clinic or treatment room and 'get it over with'. Even then, everything must be in readiness beforehand. It is cruel to start preparations having already removed the child.

HOW PARENTS FEEL

Not all parents will feel able to participate in technical procedures and this should be expected and respected. Some people cannot bear the sight of blood at any time. Others may wish to witness even the most gruesome ordeals. If one can stand aside and view each situation from the child's point of view — 'would it help if I could hold Mummy's/ Daddy's hand?' — it will be easier to make the decision.

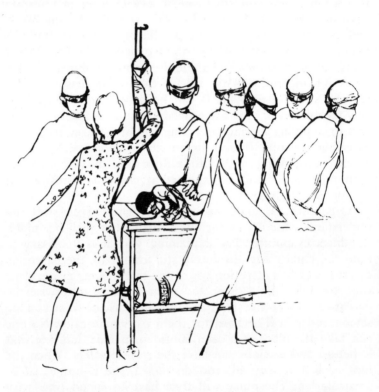

Parents will need to know what they are expected to do. It is surprising how much the very hospital atmosphere upsets the layman. I once conducted a small survey in the area around the hospital to find out what the consumer thought. What facilities did they think existed? What other things would be helpful? What were their actual reactions to their child's being in hospital? Some interesting facts emerged. The very atmosphere of the hospital was deemed to be sterile. Some mothers were confused and unsure of even knowing how to change baby's nappy. 'Because the bed is *sterile*, isn't it?' 'Where would I wash my hands?', asked another. 'Should I go into the kitchen to do so and so?' My *sterile* nurse's hands nearly shot up in horror at the thought. At the hospitals in the area this was the only room out-of-bounds to parents! The picture of the young mother looking wistfully over the side of the cot at her baby, not daring to pick him up, must be a familiar sight to all nurses. Parents may well need encouragement at the outset. They have often complained to me that no one ever told them what they could do. They may have to be shown how to cuddle the baby with a drip, how to handle an awkward frog plaster and to lift a child with sureness. Soon they are managing with as much confidence and gentleness as the best nurses. One mother managed to continue

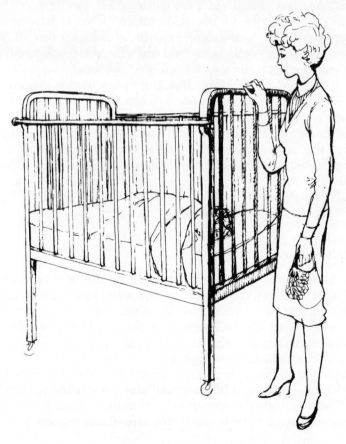

breast-feeding whilst her baby was on traction for CDH (congenital dislocation of hips).

Occasionally there are parents who, for reasons best known to themselves, suddenly decide that although they are there they do not want to help in the care of their child. In answer to the nurse's 'Would you like to wash Ann now?' comes the retort 'No, I wouldn't — what do you think you're for — it's your job, you do it.' When this sort of thing is said, it can be mortifying. It confuses the nurse and can be damaging to parental participation and family nursing. It is easy to get resentful and the nurse, rather than stifling her feelings and saying nothing, should be encouraged to report it. It will need to be understood why the parents have acted in this way. As far as the parents are concerned it can be a 'cry for help'. They may be anxious, unsure of what is happening, angry with the hospital or even their child because of his condition. They will need help and the nurse will need to be reassured that the attack is not personal in any way.

Staff need to be aware that the opposite can happen as well and needs to be resisted. When parents are available, some nurses will abdicate their responsibilities. Case family assignment should prevent this, but if the nurse is not confident she may just walk by, leaving the mother to take full responsibility for the care the child needs. This sort of neglect quickly breeds anxiety in a mother and mistrust of all the staff may develop.

THE PARENT LIAISON WORKERS OR FAMILY RECEPTIONIST

In a busy unit, it is often difficult to allocate time to explain all that one would wish to parents who come in with their children. At Northwick Park Hospital, Middlesex, there has been a unique scheme running for the last three years. There is a similar well-established scheme at the James Whitcomb Riley Hospital, Indianapolis. One member of staff has been appointed solely to look after the parents. Not only does she welcome them on admission and show them round, but is available to answer any queries and assist them in finding their way around the hospital. She also listens to them — how they feel, what concerns them, their conflicts and fears for themselves, their families and the sick child. This person is a full member of the ward team, attends reports, rounds, at liberty to speak directly to doctors and make reference when she thinks necessary to the social worker. Initially a difficult role, it has necessitated complete trust by the other members of the team, especially as she was neither a doctor nor nurse. Over the years she has established herself as indispensable, not only to the parents who know she is never too busy to listen, but also to the staff who know that so often they are too busy to listen just when the parents wish to talk. Every young houseman must have had occasions when he wearily does his last night round, only to have an anxious mother waylay him. Having waited all day to ask him some question about her child, the whole issue has become more urgent and emotionally charged in the interminable interim. With a parent liaison or family receptionist this sort of situation should be totally avoidable. Other hospitals are gradually following suit and are using a variety of personnel, nursing auxiliaries, ward hostesses in this way.

Summary

Family-centred care is so obviously the natural and best way of allowing children to receive the expert medical and nursing care they need whilst preserving for them the equally important support their families provide emotionally.

   Family-centred care is not new. The developing countries have rarely been able to admit children unless an adult comes with them to care and cook for him. In rural Africa and India, many mothers sleep either under the bed, or in bed with the child, cooking outside on the open ground. However, it is relatively new in this country. Many hospitals still regard parents living in with their children as an unnecessary luxury. Arrangements for their accommodation vary with the view taken by the staff administrators, doctors, nurses. Some facilities are elaborate, others make-shift and primitive. Few have solved all the problems associated with parents' needs. In some places, family care is such that it is possible to accommodate brothers or sisters. In some long-term hospitals, caravans have been purchased for visiting parents and in at least one hospital there is a purpose-built bungalow in the grounds which can house two visiting families.

Nurses, doctors and other ward staff are learning new skills as they work alongside parents in the care of their sick child. Parents, too, need to be given help as they learn to function within the goldfish-bowl existence of hospital life. They can also learn to handle the technological gadgetry required for the care of their child.

To cope with the many extra demands made on staff in the area of communication and counselling that parents bring, experiments are being made to allocate members of staff particularly to this role. The parent liaison worker is one that has proved successful in the last few years. This sort of imaginative caring for the whole family needs to be examined in greater depth.

Parents and family-centred care are here to stay. It is obviously in the child's interest. More efforts may be needed to provide for them but these mean expensive capital resources. There are problems for the staff and these must be faced and met too.

References

Blake, F. (1954). *The Child, His Parents and the Nurse,* Philadelphia: Lippincott.

British Paediatric Association (1974). *Planning of Hospital Children's Departments,* London.

Hales-Tooke, A. (1973). *Children in Hospital: The Parent's View,* London: Priory Press.

Haller, J.A. (1968). *The Hospitalised Child and His Family,* Oxford University Press.

MacCarthy, D. (1965). 'A Parent's Voice', *The Lancet,* 18 December 1965, 1289–1291.

Meadows, S.R. (1969). 'The Captive Mother', *Archives of Diseases of Childhood,* 44, 362–367.

Places Mentioned

Amersham General Hospital, Amersham, Bucks.
British Hospital for Mothers and Babies, Woolwich, London.

Hospital for Sick Children, Tadworth.
James Whitcomb Riley Hospital, Indianapolis, U.S.A.
Lord Mayor Trelor Hospital, Alton, Hants.
Moffatt Hospital, University of California, San Francisco.
Northwick Park Hospital, Harrow, Middlesex.
Royal Alexandra Hospital for Sick Children, Brighton.
Standford Children's Hospital, Palo Alto, California.

3 Families with Particular Needs

Introduction

To pretend that having parents on the wards, sharing in the care of their sick child, has no problems is to be unrealistic. It is my belief that the reason there are still hospitals in this country that do not include parents in all aspects of their children's care is often purely because of these very problems – both imagined and experienced.

Of course there are problems. There are families with difficulties in every community. Just because of this some of them are more likely to find themselves unable to cope with sickness in the home. It may be the result of physical and mental handicap that predisposes them to other problems – inadequate housing, poverty or marital disharmony. Under stress many people tend to react in less controlled ways. When families have a sick child the stress may be enormous. It may appear out of proportion to the degree of illness as assessed by the hospital staff. This may be due to the fears of the parents – one or other may have been sterilised and there is, therefore, no chance of replacing a precious child should he not survive his illness. The parent may have had unhappy experiences of hospital during his or her childhood, or there may be guilt that the illness of the child is somehow attributable to them. This seems to be particularly common when the child has a congenital abnormality. Burns and scalds frequently bring condemnation from the community and sometimes hospital staff so that the guilt of parents may be magnified. Young parents who feel inadequate in their handling of their child, or ignorant of things they imagine they are expected to know, may cause them to become defensive and appear aggressive at times.

Problems must therefore be expected. Moreover, there are certain types of problems that frequently arise with some categories of parent more than others. How is one to recognise potential problems and how is one to deal with them?

Broken or One-Parent Families

It is well documented that families with marital difficulties suffer from pressures which in turn can trigger off social, emotional and physical problems in the children. The broken family starts with considerable disadvantages, not least the fact that there may be only one parent, who is also the breadwinner. With the divorce rate accelerating and the number of one-parent families on the increase, it is inevitable that we must expect more child patients in this category. They are also more likely to find their way into hospital, just because of the added difficulties of caring for them in their own homes. When a child is ill, even more when a child is seriously ill, the emotional ties of parents may stimulate both parties to visit. Where the estrangement has not progressed further than the acute emotional stage, the meeting of such parents over the bed of a sick child may be exceptionally harrowing – and children may need rescuing from a confrontation at the bedside. On the other hand, it has been my experience that some children will use their illness to contrive to get the parents to visit together. One boy I knew persisted in writing to the absent parent, begging her to visit and specifying the time to come, knowing full well that the father always came at that time. The same boy exhibited, on his locker, a photo of him with both his parents in a happy family portrait.

The parents who has custody may ask that on no account shall the other parent be allowed to see the child or it may be requested that staff speak to the other parent to explain the reason the child has been admitted. More often than not, the situation arises when the least experienced staff nurse is in charge and the social worker unavailable. To have spent time listening to the parent when admitting the child, and to have established good rapport with the youngster, will pay dividends if a crisis arises. The social worker or health visitor can be alerted and clear instructions be left in case a junior mem-

ber of the nursing staff is left to handle the problem. Ideally
the arrangments should short-circuit any emotional confrontation in front of the child.

There are sadly a number of families where the second
parent shows no interest; there are also others where the
illness or death of one of the children causes marital relationships to change. Whereas some parents come together 'for the
sake of the child', there are others where the strain of seeing
a child through a lingering terminal illness is too much and
the parents separate.

Children from broken families may well need help in
expressing the fears and bewilderment they face. The play
specialist may be a tremendous help. Because of her unique
role in using materials, children often find it easier to express
themselves in play (see Chapter 9).

The Immigrant Family

Britain, like the United States and many other countries, is
now a multiracial society and there may be a need to adapt
the services of the children's ward to meet special requirements. Immigrant families bring with them the richness of
their own customs and cultures, but are often confused by
language and other differences, especially when they also
have a sick child. They pose a challenge to all who care for
them. Children from overseas may suffer from unfamiliar
diseases and may come from areas where medical care is less
sophisticated. There may be a language problem, making it
very difficult for nurses to explain the details of patient care.
Frustrations exist on both sides and sensitive efforts are
needed to bridge the cultural gaps. When the doctor has to
give such parents a diagnosis of any severity it should be given
whenever possible in the parent's language, so it may be
necessary to obtain the assistance of an interpreter. Usually
there is some member of staff working in the hospital who
can do so, otherwise there are lists of interpreters available in
the community. Where necessary the appropriate embassy will
always assist. Language cards are kept in most hospitals by
the administrators; the Red Cross also supply them. Language
cards can be invaluable in communicating simple messages

when the family do not speak English. A school-age child of the family can also help interpret but it is not always easy to explain everything through a child, especially when the child is the patient!

Whilst all of us probably still retain some concepts based on folklore medicine, many immigrant families may rely much more on such traditions. One family in my experience was terrified on learning that their son was to have radiation treatment. It finally transpired that when electricity had been introduced into their rural community back home recently, there had been a number of fatal tragedies. It was hard to believe that 'burning' as was described could have therapeutic results when skilfully used. It maybe just as bewildering when families find they are involved in isolation techniques. I knew one family whose child was suspected of cholera. We were not able to explain well enough and the mother never did understand she should not put a used bedpan on the floor outside the cubicle, or even carry it across the ward to the sluice.

Many overseas families understand better than some of us about the importance of being with a sick child. Indeed the difficulty comes when everyone wants to stay on the ward! Diet can be a problem, not only because of religious taboos

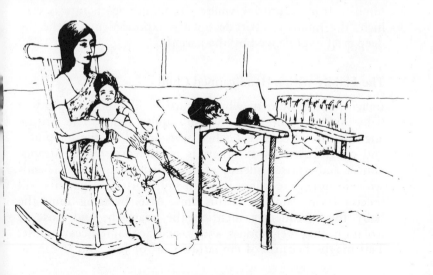

but also the unfamiliarity of the food and ways of preparing it meets with total food refusal in some fastidious and unwell youngsters. Most parents are more than happy to bring in traditional food for them. Helping them understand the restrictions of a medically ordered diet may test the ingenuity of the dietitian and may need reinforcement at ward level. For example, families from countries where Vitamin 'D' is assimilated through the action of sunlight on skin, may need to supplement their normal diet permanently. One ward sister I know has devised an illustrated chart showing the foods of various cultures that it may be necessary to exclude from a diet for say a coeliac or diabetic patient. Another chart shows good and important foodstuffs. All have captions in several languages.

Medical records have been complicated in the last few years as our traditional way of recording by 'surname' may be inappropriate to certain cultures. Families may thus be confused as to which name is required. Religion, too, may involve more cultural connotations than hospital staff expect. For instance, Sikhs do not ever cut their boys' hair. It may be important on occasions to have this sort of information should this be medically necessary. If a death occurs, it is helpful too to have some knowledge and sensitivity to various cultural ways of grieving and involvement of the extended family. In families from countries where the infant death rate is very high, the fatalistic attitude openly expressed may belie the deep grief experienced by the parents.

The Family with a Handicapped Child

Imagine for a moment what it must be like to give birth to a baby only to find that 'he isn't quite right'. The private anguish the parents feel when surrounded by the happiness and congratulations of others is made worse by the strange almost embarrassed silence of one's own relatives and friends who do not quite know what to say. Fortunate parents will receive loving support at this time. After bringing home the baby they frequently mention the heartache and sense of isolation that neighbours and casual acquaintances impose. This maybe because of embarrassment or fear, but it can be devastating to the family. Some handicaps are less obvious than others and may not be observable for some time. Parents sometimes deny their existence until comparison of their own child with his peers makes deception no longer tenable. Many parents feel guilty that in some way they are responsible for the defect. No amount of explanation or reassurance may succeed in alleviating these fears. It is extremely important that staff do not make any negative remarks in the hearing of the family. Even a remark such as 'poor little thing' can be interpreted as demeaning. However small the handicap, parents are conscious that their child is 'different'.

Not only are parents isolated in the community because of irrational fears of the neighbours, but the physical demands a handicapped child makes may leave them exhausted. When there are normal healthy children as well, conflicts may arise as to who needs the attention most. One or other is almost bound to suffer unless outside help is forthcoming. Marital disharmony can arise and it would appear there is a higher ratio of marriage breakdown in families with handicapped or terminally ill children. Certainly the reasons can be easily understood. It may be impossible for both parents ever to be free from the child who needs constant attention. Repeated visits to out-patient departments, physiotherapy or speech therapy can be an added burden on stressed parents.

Sometimes these children are regularly admitted to hospital for short periods. In this way the parents can be relieved of the full-time care and yet not relinquish their responsibility entirely. In some areas, these children spend half the week, every other week, or month, in a hospital or hostel and the alternative periods at home. Day care may also relieve the burden. Nevertheless parents sometimes feel guilty about needing relief and struggle on until their own health suffers.

When a child is in hospital it is important to remember that he too has feelings and he too will be conscious of his 'difference'.

Mandy, a little girl aged nearly five, who had had a tracheotomy for several years appeared to behave exactly as the other children. It was hard to believe that she felt different in any way. As far as she could remember she had always needed 'sucking out' and changing her tube was a regular routine. When eventually it was possible to remove the tube altogether and the site closed I wondered how she felt. Soon after, much to my surprise, she sat on my lap, stroked my throat and said 'Now I'm like you Sister, aren't I?'

Of course, not all handicapped children suffer from congenital abnormalities. Handicap may be the result of trauma, road-traffic accidents or as a direct result of disease. Parents of these children need great sensitivity and support. Particularly through the early days, they may express anger or frustration that there is no longer a chance that their ambitions for their child can be fulfilled. It can be a very hard time for the whole family. It is at this point that the skilled help of one of the specialist members of the ward team may be vital so that they are better able to adjust to the needs of their newly handicapped son or daughter.

Parents Sometimes Labelled 'Difficult'

Occasionally families are admitted who find it difficult to settle, never feel comfortable and always seem to assume that their child is not getting the care he needs. This may not be apparently serious until suddenly the tension reaches such a pitch that emotions flare up. When confronted by abuse or aggressiveness in a parent it is essential not to react sharply. How easy it is to become defensive and start justifying one's actions or those of one's colleagues. Parents may complain that everything is wrong; care is not being given on time; the child has been left in a wet bed; he has been sick and so on. How often has the nurse in charge of a baby heard this sort of complaint. 'My baby didn't have her bottle' or 'She had her last feed only two hours ago according to the food chart.' Parents who are anxious and lack trust in the hospital use any small irregularity to feed this distrust! Once someone starts looking for faults the problems magnify. Much of the factual content may be true. The anxiety it engenders inflames basic insecurity and the mother, full of fears about her baby, may become distraught.

When the husband comes to visit she spills out all her pent-up anguish on to him. Often it is the father who acts as the spokesman and he may well be reacting to the mother's anxiety superimposed on his own. There is always an enormous strain put upon parents of sick children. Guilt may be a real or imaginary factor in the parent's minds. The on-going responsibilities of the family, the pressures from relatives, even anxieties about work may be added to the gut-level emotions raised by the child's illness.

When a parent starts complaining, whether it be that the patient is being neglected or that the floors aren't cleaned, it is good to listen seriously and sensitively to what is being said. More important is to listen to what the parent is *feeling* — listening through the superficial grievances until one hears the parent's real anxiety. It may be due to failure of communication. Parents who feel left in the dark become more and more anxious and may be also aggressive. If only they felt free to ask — did my child vomit? have pain? collapse? cry? eat? It is always a cry for help. But the help needed may be the understanding of the parents' own feelings and needs.

Parents Involved in Non-Accidental Injury

Much is said today about the abused child and his parents. Very little guidance is given on how the staff in the hospital are to handle the problems these children and parents pose. Emotionally it is a volatile subject. The public gets outraged at the sight of a small child battered by an adult's uncontrolled anger. Nurses, too, when faced with caring for a badly battered child, may experience all the emotions of the community. To see the effects of such abuse and to know something of the possibilities of permanent damage that may have been inflicted makes it doubly hard not to become emotionally involved. Yet as ward doctors, nurses, paramedical staff, it is not our job to criticise, to pronounce judgement, or to become resentful. Our caring for the child will probably involve caring for the parents too. In some instances, the parent will admit to the assault; in others it is only suspected in the first instance.

Once a decision is reached to admit a child, the nurse in the casualty department has the delicate task of preparing the child and at the same time supporting the parents over this decision. She will have to convince them no one is pre-judging the issue. Despite her own feelings, she will need to accord them the same welcome as to other parents and include them in any caring task for their child. Feelings of hostility may arise and all staff need the support of the rest of the ward team if they are to be able to show understanding and compassion in their helping of the parents.

Perhaps the hardest place of all to come to terms with child abuse is in the intensive-care unit. When a child has such life-threatening injuries that it is unlikely he or she will survive without permanent physical or mental damage — if, in fact, he survives at all — the highly technical expertise of staff often takes precedence over interpersonal skills. Rarely is help offered to the staff in meeting the emotional stress caused by this sort of patient. Yet the staff may feel a sense of outrage acutely and be unable to 'accept' the brutality. Such personal distress becomes one of the hidden costs of nursing.

Although on admission it is unlikely that a firm diagnosis of abuse has been established and there may be a delay before action can be taken, whenever there is any danger that a parent may try and remove their child, a Place of Safety Order can be sought. This is most easily arranged through the social services or NSPCC. Sometimes it may have to be sought by the hospital personnel, in which case the hospital social worker will usually obtain it. The presence of an official at the serving of the Order on the parents within the hospital can make an already inadequate and insecure parent even more distrustful of the staff. However, it may be essential in some cases for the protection of the child. Equally threatening, but perhaps less recognised, is the practice of holding case conferences within the ward. Although convened there for the convenience of medical staff primarily, added tension is suffered by the parents if they become aware of such deliber-ations about their future, but are excluded from them.

Whilst in the ward the staff will find they need to be supportive towards the family: the parents may feel guilty or threatened by the hospital and perhaps by other parents who may well expect them to behave as 'model parents' and this may increase their anxiety. As often they are immature and need 'good mothering themselves' they may demand a great deal of time and patience from staff.

These parents are often particularly sensitive to what is said. Even the smallest derogatory remark by emotionally involved staff — nurses, orderlies or students — may undo painstaking work by other members of staff trying to salvage the family (see Chapters 8 and 9).

The Over-Anxious Parent

One can never assume that because the medical diagnosis on a patient is to us of a minor nature it will be seen as such by the patient or his family. One has only to remember how a septic finger can affect one's whole body and can dominate the entire day to recognise that what to medical science is minimal, to the individual concerned is a major event.

If one test result is abnormal, the parent may latch on to this to the exclusion of other good results, even though it is not important to the diagnosis or treatment. Such a mother may be swayed by other parents who are anxious and they sometimes band together to protect their babes from the *'They'*: 'You watch my child while I have a quick cuppa and then I'll watch yours.' This sort of problem can often be nipped in the bud if lines of communication are good; if parents do feel they are included and their questions truthfully answered. When a parent lacks trust in the judgement of hospital personnel, it is a small step to becoming anxious over the smallest detail. Spend time listening to the parent, especially the one who has long periods alone in a cubicle with her baby, or is separated by barrier-nursing requirements. Precious moments spent in this way may prevent tension developing.

The Young Mother and her Baby

In a busy paediatric unit it is easy to forget that young parents of a baby may in fact have never had the opportunity to learn how to handle him. They may be entirely innocent of the vagaries of their infant. In a hospital setting the advice and support of grandparents and other neighbours may be inhibited or non-existent. Breast-feeding may have been initiated, but

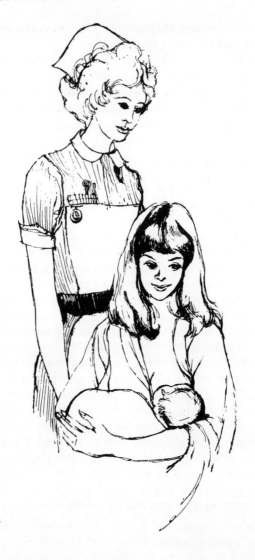

the mother may have no previous experience to help her with any of her problems. In concentrating on the ill baby, her own needs may be overlooked. When neo-nates are admitted to the paediatric wards the mothers sometimes are still 'patients' in their own right. Their midwifery needs are not always understood. The district midwives are usually most co-operative and can take over the specialised care, much as they would do in the patient's own home. It does need to be remembered, however, that often the mother is emotionally vulnerable at this time and an ill infant may cause her to be more in need of support than normal. She may feel too shy to mention her anxiety or feel so inadequate in the face of efficient nurses that she daren't. Young mothers are quick to learn and soon become highly skilled if sensitive and patient teaching is offered. When there is a liaison health visitor attached to the ward she can often build up a supportive relationship with a young mother, which will be carried over into the home on discharge.

Feeding problems are the stock-in-trade of many children's wards and the young parents bringing their babies often arrive exhausted and disillusioned. The establishment of good relationships that will be supportive and educative may hasten a satisfactory conclusion to the problems. Where the case is more complicated, such relationships will enable the ward team to stand with the parent through any necessary investigations and treatment involved, although obviously it is better if a close relationship can be established with someone such as a health visitor who is actually in the community and may be more available to advise.

Bereaved and Grieving Parents

Pehaps the most poignant and delicate of all relationships the nurse is asked to handle is when parents are told their child will not live. Often this heralds the beginning of a period of intense involvement with the family. In the case of malignant disease it may be prolonged and may ebb and flow as the child's condition runs a protracted course. In the case of accident or acute disease, it will be sudden and the family totally unprepared. It may be the final phase in a long fight with congenital handicap. It is always traumatic and the nurse must recognise this in herself. There is always a great deal that can be done and this is explained with exquisite sensitivity by Kirk's mother who writes:

When Kirk, aged 11, was first admitted to hospital Rob

and I were called into the office where the doctor and many other nursing staff were collected to tell us of the dreadful news that Kirk had leukaemia, we were assured of great support. The next day the welfare officer of the children's ward came to see me. Once again I was assured of moral support, also a visit at home was promised. No visit took place. The welfare worker concerned with very sick children should visit the home to see if housing conditions are adequate and if suitable arrangements are made for healthy children if parent or parents have to stay with the sick child.

As time went by there seemed there was a lack of contact with the doctor — no time — a rushed hello in the corridor was all Kirk and I were greeted with. I know there were other competent staff on hand to answer all our questions, but Kirk and I felt that he didn't seem interested in us anymore. If only he had made time for even once a month consultation with us. I felt Kirk was just another name on file.

My own doctor, who first told me what the first blood test showed, didn't keep in contact with Kirk. Even at the end, when I knew it was just a matter of time, once I left hospital I felt isolated. I had to cope on my own, nursing a dying child, my son Kirk, expected to nurse 24 hours a day, which I did proudly but the toll and strain showed up on me after the death.

I had to face him with a smile, pretending all wasn't so bad and cope with vomiting almost every hour of the 24 hours in the day, but then Kirk would say 'I'm sorry Mum — you go to sleep, I can manage.' He was so brave that he gave me strength that I never knew I had. I was and had to be too brave. When Kirk died I couldn't put down the brave face I had shown to him. I couldn't believe that he had gone from our lives. I really believed that he was still alive. My mind blocked — I lived like a Zombie for weeks because I had no one to relieve the pressure at home before he died.

When Kirk was first taken ill, I don't think he realised how much and how long this nasty treatment had to be inflicted upon him. Although one explains the routine, it's not the same as months and months drag on, with the same injections and terrible side effects. His confidence in me and the medical staff grew less and less. Later he refused any form of treatment after weeks of deep depression and violent tantrums and threats of suicide. This child of 11 knew he could die if treatment stopped, but Kirk was so desperate that he couldn't take any more. He was like a caged animal, pacing each room and ending in tears of deep depression. My daughter went through sheer hell. Why was she so healthy and he was so very ill. In the end Kirk terrified my daughter Jane.

It wasn't until Kirk told me he wasn't going to keep the next hospital appointment and meant it that I got through to the doctors.

I sometimes wonder if all of those weeks without treatment contributed to this. If only I had been heard with true concern and had been believed when I was pleading for the right kind of help. I have to live with this thought. Would it have made any difference if treatment had been continued?

After Kirk had died a few hours passed, then a doctor came to ask if she could carry out a post mortem. I thought he had suffered enough, but much later I thought I would have liked this, as it might have helped medical research into such cases. If this had been explained earlier I would have consented and maybe there would be more understanding what pain and discomfort is felt by the sufferer.

Kirk's mother highlights the isolation and anguish that such families experience. Often staff in the children's wards are so upset themselves when a child they have known, loved and cared for over months and sometimes years, comes to the end of his earthly life, that they are unable to help the family. There is, of course, an empathy that exists between staff and parents who care deeply about a child, but it must be remembered that unless one is able to remain objective it is impossible to support a family at the time of its greatest need. Sensitivity to the little things — time to talk, to be angry, to be inconsolably sad — all these will mean that the member of staff will need to make herself available without interruption and in a place where the parents will find it 'safe' to show their true feelings. It is not only children who feel they must be 'brave'. Parents do too, especially when the staff are doing the same thing — trying to deny the true facts, or the inevitability perhaps of approaching death. Too often medical staff will pass by the end of the bed or cubicle of a dying child during their rounds. There may be little new or positive to be reported or discussed, but the patient and the relatives are acutely sensitive to this withdrawing. Parents themselves sometimes start withdrawing towards the end of a long vigil beside a slowly deteriorating comotose child. They need a great deal of support from the staff at this time so that they do not feel guilty if they want to leave for a while. Kay's mother, a most devoted and loving one, did just this after spending weeks at the bedside. One day she told me she had spent the afternoon sitting in a deckchair in the sun. She was relieved by our encouragement and approval. It helped her when the child did die to have started picking up normal activities in her own home again.

Parents may need support for months and years after the death of a beloved child. Today there are a number of excellent self-help groups where mutual support is available. In Britain the Compassionate Friends and 'CRUSE' co-ordinate this valuable service. In the United States one of the well-known groups spreading over the country is called the 'Candle-lighters'.

Summary

To fear family involvement because of difficulties real and imagined is unnecessary, but to pretend there are no problems is unrealistic. Part of the challenge in paediatrics today is in meeting the needs of the family insofar as they affect the sick child. They are not insurmountable and the child benefits as well as the family.

There are certain problems that seem to have been magni-fied in recent years. With the rising divorce rate there are many more one-parent families bringing up their families single-handed. Acute or chronic illness will exacerbate their difficulties. Children often suffer acutely from broken marriages and on occasion have been known to try to bring about reconciliation themselves. In a similar way some children who have been victims of non-accidental injury try to prevent marital conflict. These children and their families will need sensitive and supportive loving care during the illness. Parents who are young, anxious or distrustful of hospitals, likewise will need understanding of their needs and feelings. Whatever the problem it seems the answer is to spend time to listen, to show you care and then to give any practical help that they might need. This applies as well to the grieving or bereaved parents who, because of the deep emotional wounds they have sustained, probably within the hospital itself, may need support long after the death of the child.

Whatever the sickness, whatever the need, the paediatric team should accept the challenge undaunted.

References

Burton, L., (1971). 'Cancer Children', *New Society*, 17 June 1971.

Burton, L., (ed.) (1974). *The Care of the Child Facing Death*, London: Routledge & Kegan Paul.

Burton, L. (1975). *Family Life of Sick Children*, London: Routledge & Kegan Paul.

Mitson, E., (1968). *Beyond the Shadows*, Oliphants.

Prugh, D.G., Staub, *et al.* (1953). 'A Study of the Emotional Reactions of Children and Families to Hospitalisation and Illness', *Am. Journal of Orthopsychiatry*, 23, 70.

Richardson, J., (1979). *A Death in the Family*, London: Lion Publishing.

Solnit, A.J. and Green, M. (1963). *The Pediatric Management of the Dying Child*, Part III 'The Child's Reaction to Fear of Dying: Modern Perspectives in Child Development', New York: International Universities Press, 217—228.

Voysey, M., (1975). *A Constant Burden*, London: Routledge & Kegan Paul.

Part Two

Meeting the Needs of the Whole Child

4　What is Still Important While You're Sick?

Introduction

This chapter is concerned not so much with the physical needs of sick children — food, warmth, fresh air, sleep — but with those other needs so important to their continued development, emotional and social well-being. Play, because of its priority in children's eyes, is given a chapter of its own.

When one thinks of children in a group, or even individually, one immediately gets a picture of children doing things. It may be playing with their toes if they are tiny, or even sucking their thumbs. As children become mobile they're always into something — exploring a cupboard, a handbag, surrounded by pots and pans in the kitchen. The rough and tumble of young school boys, the dressing-up of girls, playing out domestic scenes, the quiet reading of a book, painting or day-dreaming, all this is part of growing up. Children are rarely still, hardly ever unabsorbed in some activity, unless it is watching intently something that is new to them, be it the demolishing of a building, or Daddy mending the car. Thus children learn about the world in which they live, practise the skills they will need to participate in this world, and come to terms with their feelings and thoughts.

Children need to be given the opportunity to learn, not just by verbal explanation or watching, but by being included in the process. This is especially true of sick children, who, in a strange environment such as hospital, are in a totally alien world. Learning does not cease for a child just because he is sick, but he may well find it more difficult to assimilate if he is bewildered and unsure of the adults around him. Although quite young children understand what parents say, the under threes may be totally unable to comprehend the same things if said by a stranger. By entering into the child's world, it is often much easier to communicate — perhaps by using a teddy, bandages, masks, for example, in a game — and then even at this age children can understand something of what is happening to them and thus lose some of their fear. Not only do children need to be given space and opportunity to experiment and play out their experiences in hospital but also they often need to use up energy, and have certain basic needs if the normal development and growing-up process is to be continued when they are unwell.

For some children with chronic or permanent disabilities it is imperative they be given every opportunity to develop their potential. This means those caring for the sick child must make provision, not only for their physical and emotional development, but also for their educational, social and spiritual needs. These cannot be disregarded just because one is concerned with an acute paediatric ward, as there are always some patients who will need care for more than an isolated few days, and who will either become 'regulars' or who may be patients for many weeks, or even months.

The single most important need for all children in hospital is for them to be kept in touch with their families. Regular daily visiting should be the accepted norm. In many instances parents will be able to re-organise their other commitments so that one or other will be able to actually live-in with the sick child whilst he is in hospital. Where parents have long distances to travel, or inconvenient working hours, they may need advice and practical help. For older school children, friends will be very important visitors.

The Needs of Different Age Groups

One of the challenges in paediatrics is the versatility required to meet the needs of individual patients. Although there is an enormous range of differences between one child and another, there are certain guidelines differentiating the various age groups. One needs a good working knowledge of the basic stages of development, but these have to be tempered by the physical conditions and restraints the child in hospital may have.

If our aim is to meet the needs of the whole child, it is imperative we understand there are basic emotional needs of childhood. In the first year it is to be loved. This gradually develops into the awareness of belonging. This is the time for indulgence. They have to learn that mother is dependable and always there. This is when the basis of trust begins. In the second year children begin to question their own self-worth, to learn their need to be valued as individuals, for who they are, not what they do. Children of this age begin to discover there are rules. The way they are implemented, however, is very important so that children do not get the idea they are accepted only when they are doing something right. In the next few years children are concerned with their ability to perform and judge themselves according to their competence: 'I am what I can do.' It is important for caring adults to encourage and compliment children of this age — whatever their potential.

Using these as a yardstick we find our priorities for providing care for our sick children change. In some areas a radical change may be necessary.

Dr Mary Sheridan's classic work on developmental paediatrics and screening methods gives a comprehensive study of all the physical, motor and sensory stages for the under fives. Barbara Weller, in her recent book *Play for the Sick Child* (1980) has adapted these to show the types of play most appropriate for the various ages. I shall, therefore, refer only broadly to the needs of the various groups, but enough, I hope, to give a working knowledge for the staff member actually with the children. Toys children of various ages are likely to appreciate are mentioned in the following chapter.

THE UNDER ONES

Everything a baby sees, hears and feels is a new experience to him. Some babies react much more to noise than others. All respond to eye-to-eye contact and to gentle touching and cuddling. Learning from the voice and facial expression of a familiar adult (mother or mother-substitute), the baby begins to differentiate and to imitate. Babies alone in cubicles or incubators tend to get little stimulation, and conscious effort may be needed by the staff to ensure the baby is given plenty of this kind of contact. Recent research in Cambridge has shown the great difference in the weight gain of incubator babies nursed on lamb's wool mats. Might this have something to do with the caressing of the lamb's wool? As the baby learns to respond to the mother's voice, he will begin to imitate and start smiling and gurgling. He soon finds his fingers and toes and is attracted by bright colours, moving objects and those that he can catch. But remember everything is explored by putting it into his mouth. Once he begins to sit (at about six months) his world enlarges and he soon starts to initiate play himself. Its a never-ending game retrieving the toys he drops over the side of the cot or pram. Tying a long piece of string or ribbon to such a toy will enable it to be held firmly to the side of the cot without spoiling the fun of throwing it away. Once the child begins to shuffle on his bottom, look out for anything he can reach. Low-lying cupboards, examination trolleys — nothing will be sacrosanct if he is allowed to roam. If he has to remain in bed he will need plenty to occupy him, but more importantly he will want his mother. He is not yet able to play with others, but will like to have someone to initiate play with him. Before the end of the first year he will be wanting to feed himself. Try giving him a spoon and holding his hand in yours to guide him. If the process is too slow, his efforts can always be augmented by the judicious use of another spoon.

THE ONE TO THREES

A child of this age is particularly vulnerable as he may appear more independent than he really is. Adults sometimes forget that at the toddler age, the child's main need is for his mother and close family. Although it is often reported by mothers of the 18-month-old child that 'he won't let me out of his sight — I can't even go to the loo without him', he can be distraught if she disappears. Familiarity and maintenance of routine will allow him the security to explore and learn. He may be intensely curious. He will enjoy unscrewing and handling different shapes and textures of all kinds. This is the age when many children take tablets or poisons, so everything potentially dangerous must be locked and well out of reach. Some children are full of initiative and will climb to unbelievable heights to retrieve something they think mother has hidden away.

These children have little concept of time and even 'tomorrow' may be meaningless. Frustration, because he either won't or can't do something is liable to cause explosions of temper and tantrums. Fortunately it is fairly easy to divert his attention. At this stage sharing toys is not really understood and when a precious toy is snatched by another child one can expect great protestations of outrage. Truly cooperative play does not normally develop until the child is three or four. However, he will enjoy looking at picture books with others or having stories read to him.

THE FOUR TO SIX YEAR OLDS

Children now are beginning to be more worldly wise and adventurous. Some show a degree of independence from their parents whilst all is going well. They can be devastated, though, if parents are not on hand when they feel threatened, bewildered or hurt. This is the age when life is so full of wonderful things that fantasy may be indistinguishable from truth to some children with lively imaginations. Magic and imaginative playmates can be very real. Utilising the playmate can be a great help in gaining the child's cooperation. At this stage children are becoming fascinated with learning and enjoy all sorts of competition. They also begin to be aware of their own bodies. This assumes great importance as they learn more about their own identity. The fear of losing any part, however small, may be horrific, as it may threaten their self-image. The young patients need frequent reassurance that damage to one part of their body does not mean that other parts are also affected. It is particularly unfortunate when children of this age have to undergo any form of mutilating surgery, even circumcision. The fear of castration is intensified at this stage. Any discussion about operations, for example, will need great skill in order to avoid adding to their fears.

Achievement and competence in new skills are very important so they need plenty of compliments and encouragement.

Parents can be helped to do this by relaying good things you tell them their children have achieved. Certainly threats still heard 'If you're not good you'll have to stay in hospital' may prey on their young minds and unduly disturb them. As their concept of time is still limited, when visiting is infrequent, for any reason, such children may feel abandoned.

THE OVER SEVENS

This is a more independent and resilient age group. It is also one of great physical activity. Running, climbing, wrestling and all manner of communal active games are enjoyed. Increasing support comes from other children of their own age or peer groups and sometimes they show little interest in adult advice. Children over seven may suffer as much during hospitalisation as younger ones but the cause may be somewhat different. There may still be considerable dependence on parents but what friends say may matter greatly. A group of this age can get very cheeky and naughty, especially if they sense inexperience, so a young nurse or auxiliary may have a hard time and need support. Those confined to bed with orthopaedic conditions can be particularly troublesome to inexperienced new staff. Boys may find the physical restraint hard and express their frustration in belligerent or even depressed behaviour.

ADOLESCENTS

Adolescence is a no-man's-land. Not only do these young people have special needs but administratively they don't fit into the children's ward, with its accent on the needs of the very young child. Equally they are often misfits in the adult wards, which do not cater for their needs and where the other patients often see them as too noisy. It is an insecure time when many youngsters oscillate from demanding adult freedom of choice to dependence on adults for support when the going gets tough. As adolescence approaches, young patients may become self-conscious and worried about their bodies. They may cover up their fear of the future or their prognosis by means of anti-social or brash behaviour. They want and need privacy, but equally may attract noisy friends and demand loud records, seemingly deriving support and security from their presence. Irritation and intolerance of 'fussy' parents may hide the wish for their presence and support. Often the pain and anxiety of separation is just as real as with younger children. The fear of being thought 'silly', being laughed at or teased, can be intolerable.

I have found that, given the opportunity, the majority of adolescents opt for a side room in the children's ward, rather than return to the adult wards. Strangely enough, it is the boys who seem to take a real interest in the babies and younger children. More girls seem discontented with the nuisance of crying babies. Wherever they are nursed, this group of young people have definite and different needs, which should be recognised and catered for. In some progressive areas separate adolescent units are provided. The difficulty in some hospitals arises because of the relatively low numbers involved. Where they have been established the very special needs of this group have been met. Versatility of routine has been combined with a certain freedom.

In addition to the developmental needs of children, education and links with the home environment need consideration.

Education in Hospital

Some children suffering accidents or other injuries may find themselves confined to a hospital bed for a number of weeks. In some cases it may extend to months. These children will be at a serious disadvantage if their educational needs are not met. Some will be studying for examinations, others just learning to read. Whatever the stage, there are few schools with the time and motivation to help a child catch up with his classmates if the absence is prolonged. Most teachers, however, are concerned to help one of their pupils who is sick, and will provide lesson material if the parents are able to fetch this. Local education authorities are under an obligation to provide teachers for children of school age, particularly for those liable to be away from school for more than a week or so. Some authorities are able to provide specialist teachers for individual subjects, if the pupil is over 11 years old.

A few supply a regular teacher of outstanding flexibility and wide-ranging ability. When the hospital itself puts a suitable room at the disposal of the education authority it is furnished and maintained by them. In these cases, the unit is indeed fortunate. Sometimes children who have been discharged but still unable to return to school continue to attend the hospital school as 'day patients'. The variety of stimuli for the children is greatly enhanced. The teachers may work closely with the medical and nursing personnel and use contemporary experiences for their lessons. Spelling revolves round the new words learnt in hospital: maths is taught whilst measuring liquids in medicine glasses and syringes — I have even seen milk bottles filled with red liquid, obviously demonstrating a person's blood supply. Apart from this, the school and lesson routine itself can have a beneficial effect on the young patients. Where school hours can be adhered to in a flexible ward routine and specially if the children can be physically taken to school, in beds or wheelchairs where necessary, school assumes an importance by its very normality.

Links with Home

Links with home and the usual community activities that the children have can also be fostered. Traditionally, Christmas and Easter are celebrated, but so can all sorts of other occasions. Guy Fawkes Night may give rise to a difference of opinion amongst staff, but personally I feel it can be an opportunity for positive teaching about the dangers involved. But this need not preclude a firework display, complete with bonfire and guy. Even the bed-bound children have great fun helping to make the guy and often have definite ideas as to his identity, be it nurse or doctor. An occasion for a party with sausages and toffee apples, followed by a firework display, means that the patients do not feel cheated. It is also an opportunity for families to enjoy the occasion together. Doctors, porters and other staff find it a good excuse for enjoying themselves too.

Local guide companies and scout troops willingly participate by collecting for special items wanted in the wards and enjoy a visit too. Sometimes a local troop will hold a special ceremony, or enrolment, in the ward when their member is in the hospital. Sunday school can play an important role. The Salvation Army held a regular hour each Sunday in one of the wards where I worked. In another, medical students took the initiative. Both were popular and were very lively affairs. It was my experience that a number of relatives always seemed to drift over and join in, sometimes making appreciative remarks afterwards.

Although the provisions mentioned are common needs of all children, there are some patients who, because of their circumstances, deserve separate consideration.

Children with Special Needs

THE DIABETIC

Diabetics have special problems as they appear normal healthy individuals and the aim, of course, is to maintain this. Although the disease is not curable at present it should be quite possible to control — at a cost. One should not underestimate the stress imposed by daily injections and life-long dietary restrictions. Maintaining normality for the youngster, given these restraints, is not always so easy, and is sometimes a forgotten priority of nursing and medical staff. The diabetic child may be excluded from normal school activities, such as swimming, although this is quite unnecessary in most instances. He may be discriminated against in school, particularly over school meals. In one hospital I was taken to task by an adolescent girl who asked how she could be normal when we insisted that she test her urine at lunch-time. The same girl said the worst thing about diabetes was that her school friends kept asking why she had to keep missing school to 'go to the hospital' when she didn't seem ill. By changing the time of out-patient appointments, so that she could come after school, a totally new approach has been developed in this clinic. Concentrating on the needs of the child and parents everyone agrees is much more satisfactory. The children are better controlled. Some are stabilised at home and even new diabetics are no longer necessarily admitted to hospital.

By allocating the same registrar and senior nurse to all diabetic patients, whether in- or out-patients, consistent information and advice is much easier to maintain. Patients and their relatives feel free to discuss the problems as they arise. Difficulties over too rigid or restrictive a diet are avoided, and the very natural fears arising from both facts and gossip are alleviated. Liaison with schools and youth organisations have improved, as difficulties are reported when they occur and can be dealt with immediately. Some schools now issue forms for swimming instruction for example. One way better understanding of the disease has been transmitted is by using a questionnaire for parents of all new diabetics (see Appendix II). The simple facts about the disease are followed by queries: Should insulin be given if the child has been sick or not well? What about strenuous exercise? What does it matter if there's a change in pattern of urine test results? When to ask for medical help? What sort of food to give when the child is not hungry?

THE CHRONICALLY ILL CHILD

Whether he suffers from severe asthma, coeliac or congenital heart disease, eczema or cystic fibrosis, Still's disease or one of the rarer congenital conditions, he may have difficulty in keeping up with his peers. This may show itself more blatantly in low scholastic attainment and a general lack of outside interests. Such children frequently express a somewhat adult attitude towards their prognosis. Because it may be rather depressing and frankly bad in some cases, many adults tend to shrug off such topics with 'the child wouldn't understand'. Even quite young children of six or seven do understand much more often than is realised. They can be very philosophical. They can just as easily be depressed and concerned about their future or the lack of it.

By virtue of their long stays in hospital, they do sometimes become institutionalised and efforts must be maintained to keep life in the ward as normal as possible. Encouragement to be independent will aid self-confidence. Nursing children on long-term intravenous therapy or respirators will stretch the imagination of staff wanting to provide normal stimulation.

It is not impossible. For example, one baby nursed on a respirator for the first 14 months not only learnt to crawl, but enjoyed a daily bath in the sink like anyone else. Older children have been taken shopping and spent regular times out-of-doors. Happily there are now very few children for whom hospital must be 'home'. Modern drugs and improved operative procedures have changed all this. Those receiving such care tend to be those with multiple handicaps usually associated with some degree of mental incapacity. It is now strongly recommended that these children receive family-type care such as is provided through the social services. Where hospital care is essential, it is further recommended that the staff are trained in child care, rather than concentrating on nursing techniques alone. Services are beginning to be provided in the community so that families can share the care of their handicapped youngster with professionals. Day care, weekly care and places such as Honeylands in Devon, where support is flexible, can meet the need of individual families.

At the Jewish Hospital Denver, Colorado, specialising in long-stay children with respiratory disease, the traditional wards have been adapted to make small living groups in charge of house parents, rather than nurses. The children have bedrooms with bunk beds, and help to prepare their food and care for their clothes. They progress to being totally responsible for their own routine drugs, even to setting alarm clocks for night medication. The change was proving of great benefit to often seriously disabled and chronically sick children and made it much easier for their eventual rehabilitation, I was told when I visited.

THE PHYSICALLY HANDICAPPED

In an acute paediatric ward the staff may feel apprehensive of severely handicapped children, especially if they have a prosthesis or complex aids. When these children are to be hospitalised for short periods, staff tend to do everything for them, as time is limited and it is quicker. Staff are often unaware that seemingly helpless children can, in fact, do a great deal. The parent, teacher or school nurse will be able to help as they have been party to the long struggle towards independence. When there is a prosthesis, a member of the paediatric staff should never mind admitting that she is unfamiliar with it. Neglect of its proper care may cause the child weeks of later agony if a pressure sore develops owing to its incorrect alignment or maintenance. Apart from their physical requirements, staff will want to know ways in which these children can enter the activities of the group. As suggested in the chapter on play, it may be possible to adapt the height of tables so that children in a wheelchair can participate with their peers. One of the more difficult problems is giving these children means by which they can become independent.

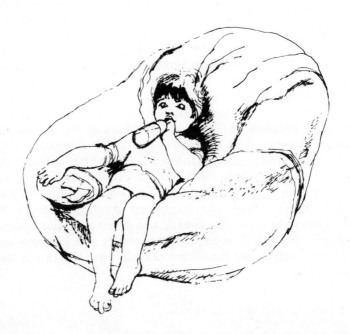

They are often determined to do everything and it is sometimes difficult to know when they must be restrained for their own safety, and when they should be allowed to try. Wheelchairs today are greatly improved and even miniature models are electrified. Low trolleys, with outsize rubber tyres, have been designed by the Spina bifida association and mean that floor games can be enjoyed. I saw one normal-height trolley

adapted with bicycle wheels so that an adolescent boy, confined to lying prone because of severe spinal problems, could
be mobile. He became the hospital messenger with obvious
joy and satisfaction. The children become very competent,
despite their handicaps, but beware lest they enter the
'dangerous driver' category by hurtling round the ward.

For children in full-length plaster of Paris casts, and little
ones in frog plasters, mobility can be given by platforms on
shepherd casters on which they may soon learn to whizz
around. Some children who are spastic or quadraplegic find
tremendous enjoyment when laid on water beds or small
trampolines, where the slightest movement is transmitted and
exaggerated. Inflatables and outsize soft toys are other suitable forms of apparatus for the children's use.

When the physical handicap is severe, speech may be almost
impossible. A relatively new form of communication has been
devised in Canada. The 'Bliss System' of outlines (a type of
picture shorthand) is portrayed on a board, sometimes clipped
on to the child's wheelchair. By division into sections for
nouns, verbs and certain phrases, children who were previously
ignored for their seeming lack of intelligence are now able to
communicate, ask for what they want, explain feelings and
make comments. Sometimes it is a painstaking process as the
child may be able to point only with his eye; others may have
the use of fingers, hands etc. Some can use pointers attached
to their foreheads by headbands. One boy of ten, about to be
admitted to hospital from school, indicated to the nurse that
he wanted to take his electric wheelchair with him. The nurse,
frankly, was sceptical but latter admitted he was right and
the chair was invaluable to him. She used this illustration to
show the way in which the system was able to improve the
life style for the grossly handicapped child, who normally
had no way of communicating. There are other non-verbal
systems of communication but they require some manual
dexterity. They are used with some success with the mentally
handicapped.

Because of their restriction, it is only recently that attention
has been directed to these children receiving everyday experiences. Going by bus, shopping, making telephone calls and
washing up.

CHILDREN WITH NON-ACCIDENTAL INJURIES

It must be remembered that most children subject to non-accidental injury are not unloved children. They very often have had good experiences within their families. Some are brave enough to stand between their rowing parents and try on their own to solve marital conflict; others have an immature and isolated parent, who herself needs good parenting and who has never learned to handle stress.

But when children have been subject to long periods of abuse, they may be fearful of adults and cower if reprimanded. Some are hyperactive, undisciplined children who, like their parents, are victims of their own emotions. More than hospital care, these children usually need a period of stable calm and consistent handling from a small team of loving mature adults (preferably only one or two), who may or may not be working with the family. They may need assessment as to their psychological damage and may also require physical building-up. Some inevitably have the added burden of prolonged neglect or serious physical injury. These children may never have built up any meaningful relationships and be emotionally damaged.

Although most abused children are admitted initially to hospital for assessment and diagnosis, a number remain for some weeks or even months whilst social service administrators and magistrates deliberate about their future. Wherever possible they should be moved quickly to a more normal environment, where the routine and discipline is geared to healthy children and not sick ones. It is also difficult to help the parents of these children within an acute ward scene as they often require much time and support. From the parents' point of view hospital, on the other hand, can be a safe and acceptable place which does not immediately condemn them in the eyes of the community. A great deal of local support and sympathy is offered to a family whose child is taken to hospital, and although it may initially help to soften the blow, the parents may meet antagonism from other parents in the ward if the reason for admission becomes known. Visiting may be stressful for them, as other visitors, not knowing the circumstances, may expect them to behave as 'good parents'.

The staff may need to give them more time, help and support than they would normally lavish on the child. This will be part of their care.

CHILDREN WITH KIDNEY FAILURE

These children are very much aware that they live precarious lives. They may have fantasies about the dialysis machines, their shunts and especially about blood. They are understandably preoccupied with their chance of getting a transplant and at times will revolt against the seemingly interminable routine. Some children to whom I have spoken have complained mostly about the restriction of diet and particularly the low ration of fluids. In one or two units the end of the dialysis is celebrated with an unrestricted meal which the children plan and anticipate whilst they are attached to the kidney machine.

Depression and general malaise is a common feature and those caring for such children need great sensitivity in knowing how and when to encourage them to be active and when to sit and listen is the best course. The Child Study Center Yale published a case study on one adolescent child who refused further treatment, choosing rather to die, which she did, but with the consent and understanding of family and staff. Staff come to know these children very well as they are regular attenders in the unit. It is sometimes difficult to remain objective, especially when things go wrong and the staff need a great deal of support themselves.

The children get to know each other well and follow each other's progress. Now that many will be candidates for a transplant the older child, particularly the adolescent, is bound to have deep feelings about his chances, as well as those of the transplant recipient. Usually there is a psychiatrist attached to the unit to help with the problems but all members of the team must be sensitive to their need to talk, act out their feelings and to express anger with their own bodies. The teacher may be the chosen confidante as she is a little less involved with the technical side and often represents the normal outside 'real world'.

TERMINALLY ILL OR DYING CHILD

The dying child and his family pose problems at a deep level, and provide perhaps the ultimate in demands on the skill and caring of the ward staff. Somehow humans revolt at the idea of a child dying. The elderly, for whom death has slowly approached in the fulness of time, may be accepted and there has hardly been time for a neo-nate to establish deep ties with the family, but when a growing child with the future before him dies, civilised man is appalled. Children do not always seem to view death as adults do. Some older children get depressed and fearful, others do not seem to suffer in the same way. Dr Bluebond-Langner, in her sensitive research contained in *The Private Worlds of Dying Children* (1979),

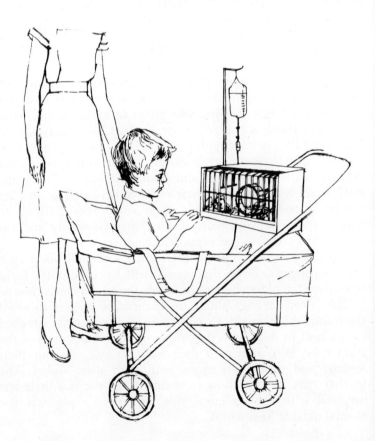

shows they do go through certain recognised stages of growing realisation.

The main need for the dying child is, I think, for the staff to become sensitively aware of his feelings, to be truthful in any information or answers given and, above all, to have time to listen to what the child wants to say. It is fatally easy to change the subject when the words are painful to hear. No one likes to think of a child suffering — let alone knowing he is dying. Nurses and doctors have traditionally protected themselves from such conversations with adults by showing a cheerful 'You'll feel better tomorrow' attitude. Instead, listen very carefully to children when they start to talk. It is not always necessary or wise to answer a question too quickly or glibly — it may well stop further conversation. Try turning the question round and repeating it back to the child 'So you think . . . do you?' Be prepared to wait for many minutes, if necessary. If you're relaxed, the child will gain confidence. Too often children have to put on a brave front, particularly with their parents, and do not let on how they are really feeling. What an indictment if they have to do the same with the nurse and doctors.

Even children very near to death may be determined to continue normal life. They will want to watch their favourite television or pop star — and possibly as loudly as ever! One boy recently was adamant he was going to sit his 'O' levels. He did complete them and after his death his parents found he had passed them all. By the judicious use of drugs, one small boy of four, dying of lymphosarcoma, was able to live and play at home and as he was happy gave his parents great comfort in his last weeks. Because children are so sensitive to atmosphere, it is imperative that parents and staff agree about their handling of the patient. If normal discipline is totally abandoned, or the child given into over every whim, life may become unbearable for the staff and parents, especially if life is prolonged. On the other hand, the family may feel guilty and reproach themselves if the child dies and they have denied him even the slightest pleasure. Consistency will give the child the greatest comfort and support. One needs also to be aware of the things that are important to the child. One boy of 12 I knew, who had a wig after chemo-therapy had caused his hair to fall out, was so anxious lest his sister or friends should discover his 'awful secret' that he insisted on sleeping and bathing in it. He refused to enter any outside game or go swimming for the same reason.

Alternatively, a 13-year-old girl, although fitted with an attractive wig, refused to wear it at all. She felt it made her look different.

When it is known chemo-therapy of this nature is to be used, it is a good idea to order the wig in good time so it is available as soon as it is needed. It is also easier to obtain a good likeness. The embarrassment of a wig or the steroid-induced bloating of the body 'like a Michelin man' may be far more intolerable than the more serious implication of the disease process.

THE UNCONSCIOUS CHILD

No discussion on the specific needs of certain children is complete without mention of the unconscious child. Although students are taught to approach all patients as if they could hear and understand, it is pertinent to remind ourselves of this with the unconscious youngster. Parents can be encouraged to keep stimulating their child by talking about home, general activities and any special interest they may know he has. One little boy of six I nursed for many weeks made his first conscious movement in response to his favourite record. A 12-year-old boy, badly injured in a road accident, was completely unresponsive for four months. His family gave him daily bulletins on the family activities, his school friends visited, chatting around his bed; there was even a birthday celebrated over his inert body. Little wonder that when he did regain consciousness he seemed to be quite in touch with reality. As he improved, he was able to report all sorts of things he 'remembered' from that time when no one else was aware he could hear, let alone understand. We can never be sure but we should never presume.

Summary

For children in hospital it cannot be assumed that the provision of good physical care, of however high a standard, is sufficient to meet the needs of the whole child. Wherever sick children are accommodated, it is essential that their other needs are considered. First and foremost will be the need for the child to be kept in as close touch as possible with his parents, family and friends by regular visiting, even if parents cannot live in. The decision about how much and how often this contact is maintained should be determined by the parents and not by any restriction imposed by the hospital. Although all children will need to play, to learn, they also need support emotionally and spiritually. They need to be kept in touch with the community and with the activities of their peers.

Children with certain diseases have specific needs and these must be met by paediatric staff. Recognition of their feelings and a readiness to listen will be of more value than elaborate equipment. Much can be done to alleviate the trauma of sick children coming to terms with their handicaps if staff are sensitive to the peculiar difficulties these children face in an adult-orientated world.

The art of communication and the importance of play and its value to the sick children are a subject in themselves. Some hints for suitable materials and methods found to be acceptable in paediatric practice are discussed in later chapters.

References

Bax, M. and Bernal, J. (1974). *Your Child's First Five Years,* London: Heinemann Health Books.

Bluebond-Langner, M. (1978). *The Private Worlds of Dying Children,* New Haven: Princeton University Press.

Brazelton, T.B. (1969). *Infants and Mothers: Differences in Development,* Dell Publishing Co.

Burton, L. (1971). 'Cancer Children', *New Society,* 17 June 1971.

Burton, L. (1974). *Child Facing Death,* London and Boston: Routledge & Kegan Paul.

Burton, L. (1975). *Family Life of Sick Children,* London: Routledge & Kegan Paul.

Homan, W. (1969). New York: *Basic Books.*

Homan, W. (1970). *Child Sense,* London: Thomas Nelson.

Illingworth, R.S. (1972). *The Development of the Infant and Young Child* (5th edn), Baltimore: Williams & Wilkins.

Jolly, H. (1975). *Book of Child Care,* London: George Allen & Unwin.

Leach, P. (1977). *Baby and Child,* London: Michael Joseph.

Ministry of Education (1961). *Education of Patients in Hospital,* Circular 312.

Petrillo, M. and Sanger, S. (1972). *The Emotional Care of the Hospitalised Child:* Philadelphia: Lippincott.

Pill, R. (1977). *The Long-Stay Child Patient,* occasional paper, *The Nursing Times,* 7.7.72.

Pillitteri, A. (1977). *Nursing Care of the Growing Family,* Boston: Little, Brown & Co.

Plank, E.N. (1962). *Working with Children in Hospitals,* Cleveland: The Press of Case-Western Reserve.

Provence, S. and Lipton, R.G. (1962). *Infants in Institutions,* New York: International Universities Press.

Savage, J.H. (1975). 'The Red Arrow', *The Nursing Times,* 20 Nov. 1975.

Sheridan, M.D. (1967). *The Developmental Progress of Infants and Young Children,* London: HMSO.

Solnit, A.J. and Green, M. (1963). *The Paediatric Management of the Dying Child,* Part III 'The Child's Reaction to Fear of Dying.' *Modern Perspectives in Child Development,* New York: International Universities Press, 217–227.

Weller, B. (1980). *Helping Sick Children Play,* London: Ballière Tindall.

Places Mentioned

Child Study Centre, Yale.
Children's Hospital, Phoenix, Arizona.
Children's Hospital, Washington.
National Jewish Hospital, Denver, Colorado.
National Treatment Center for Child Abuse, Denver, Colorado.
University Hospital, Denver, Colorado.

Addresses

CRUSE: Cruse House, Sheen Road, Richmond, Surrey.
Society for Compassionate Friends: Mrs C. Mann, 25 Kingsdown Parade, Bristol BS6 5UE.

5 Play

Introduction

In meeting the whole needs of the child, play must obviously be included. Whole books have been written on this subject, and at least three especially on play for children in hospital. Because of this, I shall limit this section on play to those principles which I believe essential to our understanding of the child's need to play and to the practical implications of this in hospital.

Parents sometimes offer to give to hospitals, or ask advice as to what toys are needed. I have, therefore, included a selection of play materials that I have found acceptable to patients and staff, especially to children with specific needs. In units where one is fortunate enough to have good teaching

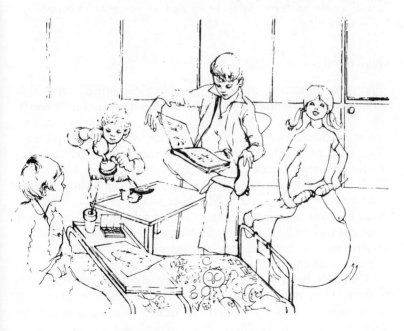

staff and an experienced play specialist, these suggestions may appear superfluous, but there are always times and occasions when neither of these invaluable members of the ward team are available and there are children crying out for 'something to do'. A minimum of equipment – paper, paste and scissors – may be quite enough to stimulate imaginative play, especially if augmented by discarded items of everyday ward life. One child of three spends happy hours under her cot scrubbing with her hairbrush and an empty 'Squeezy' bottle.

For children, play is far more than fun, diversion, or even occupational therapy. Some describe it as the child's work. Certainly it is a vital part of development. Susan Harvey in her book *Play in Hospital* (1972) says: 'Deprived of play, the child is a prisoner, shut off from all that makes life real and meaningful. Play is not merely a means of learning the skills of daily living. The impulse to create and achieve, working through play allows the child to grow in body and mind. Play is one of the ways in which a child may develop a capacity to deal with the stresses and strains of life as they press upon him. It acts, too, as a safety valve, allowing him to re-live and often come to terms with fears and anxieties which become overwhelming.'

Play for the Sick Child?

Play has particular meaning to those concerned with sick children, as it helps to maintain and restore a child's confidence in himself. It can be one of the most useful tools to assist in the recovery and rehabilitation of the young patient. The wise physiotherapist will find breathing exercises much easier if she produces a table tennis ball and plays 'blow football', or has a race blowing bubbles with the younger ones. For years mothers have used games in the bath, or fed teddy his dinner as an encouragement to the reluctant child. Nurses and doctors will find precious moments spent playing before attempting an examination or treatment will save upset, prevent lack of cooperation and often save time.

Children need to be able to play alone, as well as with others. They need privacy and somewhere to hide. They also need space. The sick child will be fickle. Whereas in health he may show concentration on one activity for considerable lengths of time, sickness, malaise, discomfort or typical restriction may mean he cannot persevere even at his favourite game for more than a few moments. His tastes may be more juvenile, his manner totally out of character. Children can become depressed and aggressive when frustrated by illness. Even the most independent child may welcome initiative and encouragement by an adult, especially if she is patient. Having a story read can be very soothing; watching other children play a good alternative to participation when energy is lacking. Children who are too ill to play do not always want to be shut away quietly — they often elect to be taken into the playroom 'to watch'. Even the sickest will ask for the radio or television. Quietness is the most common criticism of children returning from adult wards, or intensive-care units.

Music can be much appreciated too. Group efforts to produce a band may sound awful but may be much enjoyed. An old piano is sometimes donated and in the playroom, away from the acutely ill, it can be most popular.

Suitable Play Materials for Sick Children

There are such enormous differences between one child and another, regardless of age, that it is difficult to make provision for well children of every age group. Because of the short attention span of sick children and the large age range in the average paediatric unit, it must be acknowledged that one can never have too much! Toys are expensive. They tend to get lost or broken. Some are specific to a small group of children and therefore may be regarded as an extravagance. Well-wishers sometimes offer to bring or buy toys for the children's ward. It is good to keep in the back of your mind the sort of play equipment that 'someone someday might give you'. Large musical instruments such as a glockenspeil will give endless pleasure to a large variety of children, yet it is unlikely that ordinary ward funds can be spared to buy one.

A large rocking horse is, in my opinion, by far the best ambassador for any children's ward. By putting it in a prominent position near the entrance, or sister's desk, new apprehensive patients are diverted from the unfamiliar sights and sounds. Viewed from astride the horse, they can be faced with greater calm and objectivity. Another 'must' I think, is a sturdy Wendy house. Being shut away inside gives many children the hiding place and privacy they seek. These I have seen adapted as children's hospital houses and with the help of volunteer carpenters, child-size trolleys, beds and charts can be made. With cut-down gowns, discarded stethoscopes, masks, spatulae, children spend hours 'operating' and playing out their own particular brand of hospital life (see p. 115).

Apart from a 'hospital' corner (or adapted Wendy house) a home corner is appreciated by a large age range. To be able to play with familiar items bridges the gap between home and hospital that can be so painful for the child patient. A sink, a stove and ironing board, again may be able to be made by volunteers. In one unit where I worked we had an indefatigable inventor-engineer, who not only made marvellous mechanical adaptations for medical equipment, but also turned his hand to more familiar things. By far the most popular was the true-to-life scale model of a telephone kiosk. Cooking real food is always popular, but play dough and pastry making is an acceptable alternative. Sand and water play is welcomed by a large age range.

PETS

A fish tank is a marvellous acquisition for a children's ward. If it can be placed near enough for an ill child to watch or, even better, if a mobile tank can be made, it can then be taken to the child's bedside or cubicle. In one intensive-care unit I visited, a mobile fish tank had been found to be far more popular than television.

Animals provide living, moving contact for those confined to bed and unable to have normal tactile experience. For many children in bed, the only touching is by others, by washing or nursing procedures. It can be therapeutic for such children to have a rabbit or hamster playing on the bed with him for short periods. In a few units, where they are more ambitious, there is a ward dog, or even a donkey or two, who live in the outside playground. I have personally found that, in a few instances, being able to admit a small pet with the child has made a tremendous difference to him. Certainly visiting by favourite pets is sometimes more popular and comforting than by relatives!

OUTSIDE PLAY AREAS

Children asked about their feelings whilst in hospital often complain they miss going out of doors. Children find it very hard to have to stay in bed, and even harder, to stay indoors. In the majority of hospitals, access to the grounds is not an impossibility. More often it is complicated because these are some distance from the ward, and possibly on another level. Shortage of staff may preclude patients from being taken outside, but often the idea of moving beds outside is never considered. In the warm weather, it is most therapeutic to get patients outside, even in their beds. Why not have lunch outside too? A picnic can be a real treat, and parents are willing runners.

Fortunately, children's wards tend to have periods when they are not too busy, and these are the times such outlandish ideas can be put into practice, even for the acute wards. If an outside area can be reserved for the children, it may be possible to persuade a local organisation to raise money for equipment. A sandpit, a climbing frame (though not a see-saw because of the dangers, please) may be purchased in this way, but do make sure the area is protected against traffic. Space-hoppers, badminton rackets and shuttlecocks, toy barrels and, of course, a football and tricycles, toy motor cars or tractors will be prized. If you acquire a small paddling pool, it will need to be closely supervised, as accidents happen quickly, even in small amounts of water and it must always be emptied immediately after use.

INDIVIDUAL TOYS

Games, jig-saws and complicated construction toys need a great deal of care. The loss of just one small part can render the whole game useless. 'Lego' and building toys are so popular that one can never have too much. Indestructible toys, such as the 'Fisher-Price' range and the 'Play People' are also good stand-bys as they allow children to invent their own games round the figures. Paper, paint, glue, felt-tip pens and scissors provide endless variety for all ages and can be used whether the child is mobile, bedfast or isolated. Miniature toys, such as farms, zoos and dolls' houses and furniture, are also acceptable.

A large dolls' house hospital, as described by Madeleine Petrillo (1972), can be made from discarded domestic items and can be therapeutic as well as attractive to children up to adolescence.

I have found that, by keeping a private store of one or two special toys, when there is a particularly distressed child or a very lonely isolated youngster, the beautifully dressed doll or the wind-up garage is available to meet their urgent need. Once these items get into the general supply, they will have a short effective life, so it's worth keeping a few tucked away for such emergencies.

A box of dolls' clothes, a doctor's bag, the nurse's uniform, are marvellous bed toys. Some units keep 'comfort bags', brightly coloured bags containing a selection of small and different articles and toys, somewhat along the lines of a Christmas stocking. These may be given out to a new or unhappy patient.

SPECIALLY FOR BABIES

For the baby, mobiles both handmade and purchased, are available in great variety. Many are brightly coloured and catch the light; others have musical boxes attached. Rattles, rings, bells, wooden spoons and a selection of different textures can be hung across the cot. Babies put everything in their mouths, so the playthings need to be able to be disinfected if used by more than one. Plastic mirrors are a source of great interest and, for the older baby, there are more sophisticated cot toys with a variety of knobs, handles and bells to interest and intrigue. Don't forget that even young babies appreciate music and singing nursery rhymes or lullabys are part of the tender loving care that goes with a cuddle after feeding. Once babies start to kick, turn over and crawl they will appreciate a change of scene. A blanket in a safe corner of the ward or in a playpen will provide good 'kicking space'. As the toddler age is reached, their play area may need some protection from older, more robust, active youngsters who inadvertently may bowl them over.

Sick Children's Special Needs

Little has been said specifically about painting and drawing; using authentic equipment to play hospitals has been alluded to. These two activities, more perhaps than any others, help children to come to terms with the often frightening experiences that every patient meets. One 11-year-old boy, who had recently been diagnosed a diabetic, covered sheets and sheets of paper with cemeteries, crosses and spectre-like beings. The colours were uniformly black and red. There seemed to be a recurring theme of knives dripping blood. Another nine-year-old boy drew a spidery but detailed drawing of a headless man with a surgeon's knife and cutlass-like scalpel dripping blood. The head was lying nonchalantly at the bottom corner of the paper. This boy was due to have a spitz-holter valve inserted later that day. We thought he had understood how it was to be done! A photograph caught this lad in the act and he looked up with a huge grin from rapt concentration on his masterpiece. On another occasion, a young girl of 11, who had a lot of bother with a phrenic abscess following appendicectomy, painted a life-like green foetus, which she subsequently was able to talk about in relation to her fears and feelings. Not all paintings are this dramatic, but may be equally satisfying to the child patients.

'HOSPITAL' PLAY

The use of hospital equipment — stethoscopes, syringes, bandages, even masks – allows children endless variety to play out their own feelings in a symbolic way. Whether they are just available for spontaneous play in an adapted Wendy house, or offered by the play specialist, together with a doll or teddy to act as a patient, they are welcomed by the children. In some units that I know there are definite 'Play' hospital sessions, but these should not be undertaken without skilled staff and a good knowledge of the patients and the unit. Even more sophisticated medical equipment is then made available and staff volunteers act as patients. Once I observed two young boys become very excited in their play. One picked up the largest syringe he could find and started aggressively to 'inject' the patient's head (he was a doctor volunteer) — then his eye. A great deal of feeling went into this procedure and was accompanied by obvious glee. I later learnt that this boy had severe asthma and had often needed intravenous injections. In another unit, which specialised in adolescent care, the sessions were found to be a real outlet for emotional feelings. Reports of improved behaviour followed such sessions.

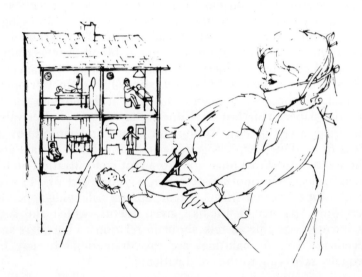

More frequently, staff playing with or alongside children, find conversations tend to be about the feelings and fears the children have over their own bodies and what has happened. It is surprising how differently children may think. The classic example must be of the child who confided after a squint operation that he was lucky because he got his own eye back, and you could never be sure when the doctor took the eyes out that you wouldn't get someone else's by mistake! The use of dolls in explaining procedures to the young patient is further discussed in Chapter 6.

Needs of Children with Specific Problems

DISABLED CHILDREN

For the handicapped child, there is added the frustration that he is unable to use some or all of the exciting toys in the ward. If he is confined to a wheelchair, for example, he will not be able to reach the floor. Many other activities may be at the wrong height. Try getting a water trough or sand tray put on table legs that allow a wheelchair to get underneath the edge. At least one table in the play-room needs to be of this height too. A punch ball hung above the bed, or between two wheelchairs, for example, may encourage a letting-off steam in a positive and satisfying manner. Often the disabled child will be too handicapped to be able to make use of these toys. Putting a multiply-handicapped child on a large sag-bag may allow him to feel included in the play circle, and yet be comfortably supported by the flexibility of the cushion. Out-

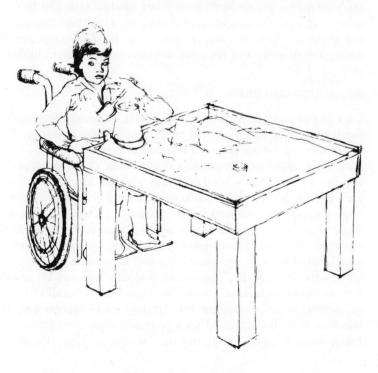

size teddies can be used, providing the child isn't too athetoid in his movements. Mobiles hung from the ceiling and the judiciously placed long mirrors are also effective. Grababiles which have toys rather than fragile items and are hung at a child's reaching height can be much more satisfying. Toy libraries often specialise in toys suitable for the handicapped. They will often help out, even if the child is in hospital.

ENERGETIC CHILDREN

Perhaps the most difficult need to meet in a confined general-hospital environment is for children to let off steam. Ward life is bound to be constricting and there is little space for children to run about in the normal way. As the majority of children today are not confined to bed even in acute paediatric wards, they will naturally want to rush about at times. Long corridors become racing tracks if one is not careful. It is for these children that an outdoor area is so helpful. Individual children are pleased to accompany a member of staff who has to visit other parts of the hospital, and may go with their parents to the shop or canteen if their condition allows. Group games, acting, dressing-up and music all help to occupy active children.

BED-BOUND CHILDREN

Except for not being able to run about, it should be possible for the bedfast to enter into most other ward activities. The possibility of being wheeled outside is one, moving into the playroom, especially for meals if the other children eat there and being 'taken' to school each day gives an air of normality. This is why I consider it so important that the schoolroom is large enough to take bed-bound patients. Often it is only the door that is too small! Even when children have old beds elevated because of traction, it is possible to obtain a device which satisfactorily elevates the mattress without raising the wheels from the floor. This means that the beds can be moved just as easily as normal ones. Try transferring small children to prams so they can be moved easily. Those on gallows traction may be attached to a portable apparatus and so be taken outside, even shopping in the pram. (This effectively means that most of the small children should be able to be nursed at home.)

Water play can be very satisfying too. Great fun can be had with funnels and transparent tubing, especially if the water is coloured with powder paints. This will, of course, need supervision and help. Little ones like to wash clothes and in certain circumstances sand trays can also be put on beds, but it is not recommended if the child is in plaster or has had eye surgery. Where it is possible, a young sibling or baby held carefully on the bed can give that contact with a living, moving being discussed in a previous paragraph. By putting two children's beds together, board games, or even table football, can be enjoyed. Any creative activity, such as watching plants grow (mustard and cress) is very easy and so are carrot tops, or cooking is much appreciated. Cakes and biscuit mixes are a boon if there is access to an oven for cooking.

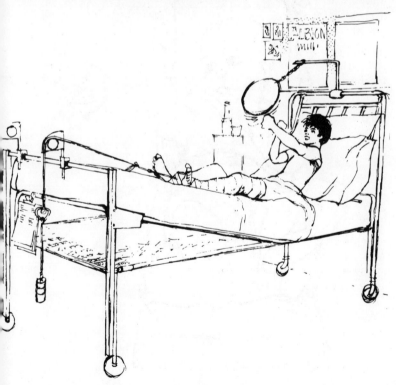

ISOLATED·CHILDREN

Isolation and barrier nursing pose very special problems for staff and patients alike. No one enjoys the prospect of being cut off from the rest of the world—even when one's world is only a ward. When barrier nurse technique is added, patients sometimes say they feel contaminated, like lepers, unclean. Every member of staff with responsibility for such children needs to be acutely aware of the effect such procedures have on their patients (see Chapter 8). Special effort must be made

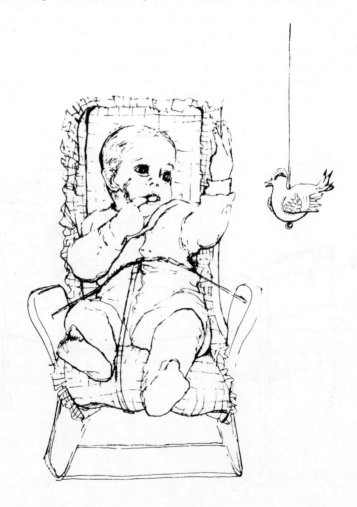

to alleviate the distress and make the child feel wanted and included. These children, more than others, need someone with them. Yet they are the most often alone. They have fewer visitors, the staff stay away, and ward activity too often goes on in apparent silence outside the glass partitions. Intercom telephones, portable televisions, activities initiated by the play specialist and nurses between children in adjoining cubicles, all can help to lessen the isolation. I have heard that some children manage to play games between cubicles by having their beds put against the separating window. If these children can be allowed to grow plants, continue with their schoolwork and so on this may all help to keep them in touch with normality. As these children, more than any others, will want to see out of the window, it might be possible to raise the bed height or move it so this is possible. In some places a bird table or coconut can be hung within view so the child can watch. Keeping some special easily disinfected toys for children in isolation will ensure staff always have something to offer a bored or homesick patient.

In some units, tiny babies are nursed in cubicles and therefore effectively in isolation. It is good to remember that these babies need stimulation too. Often the cubicles are all but soundproof. Music, singing, crooning will help stimulate the baby. Some units use the ward radio or even transistors but they are very impersonal. A rocking chair will encourage the adult, parent or staff to relax and cuddle the babe (see p. 35).

THE VERY SICK AND TERMINALLY ILL CHILD

As mentioned earlier, very sick children like to be included in the ward activities, and will ask to be wheeled to the playroom — even when they cannot participate. Passive playing, listening to stories, watching television and having their own cassettes may be the most acceptable forms of entertainment. Don't forget, though, that to be artificially cheerful, pretending all will be well in a few days, may be bolstering your morale, but not the child's. Rather than play, your young patient may have some serious questioning to do, and it may be you that he feels will give him a truthful answer. This is further discussed in Chapter 4.

Staff Involvement

In an increasing number of paediatric wards and certainly in most of the larger units, there are now play specialists and nursery nurses, whose responsibility it is to organise and supervise play (see Chapter 9). They are invaluable and are often the most missed, both by patients and staff. To the child, it is imperative that play is not fragmented because of a myriad of other duties, but is geared to the mood of the moment. Another important part of the play specialist's job is the maintenance of equipment. A box of toys, a cupboardful of games and shelves of comics are more than likely to contain only armless dolls, or wheel-less cars, missing jig-saws and tattered incomplete stories or comics. Even a game of Monopoly is no good without the dice. Remember that a firm board or table makes many games and activities much easier. In one large hospital I visited in the United States, a full-time handy man was employed to mend toys! Maybe we should take note of this idea. Too often expensive toys are discarded because there is no one willing to effect necessary repairs.

Whether or not play staff are employed, every member of the ward team needs to know how to initiate and use play. Nurses, perhaps most of all, will find play an invaluable tool in their contacts with children of all ages. Bath-time can and should be fun for everyone. In the next chapter, its role in communication is discussed. Once one has become used to 'using' play it is almost inconceivable that one could manage without it. Once ward staff have experienced organised play sessions, there is an outcry if these are suddenly withdrawn, do not function at evenings and weekends, or over holiday periods. Sometimes it is possible to stagger the hours play staff work, particularly if there are more than one in the ward. Volunteers are of tremendous value, but it is difficult for them to organise an on-going programme, as they come less often than the full-time staff, perhaps only once or twice a week. Maintenance of equipment may then become a problem. One children's ward I know does have a most successful play group run entirely by volunteers with the co-operation of social services and the Pre-school Playgroups Association.

The ward sister is very committed and is able to find the time to act as co-ordinator, but not many units, I think, will be able to do this.

Summary

Play is not an optional activity but a vital part of normal development of children. No person caring for children can ignore its importance. Sick children need play just as much as their more healthy companions. In some ways their needs in play will differ and the play may be more significant.

As children come to terms with the trauma of hospital and even the sickness itself, play may be the only medium through which the child can face the facts and express his feelings about them.

The provision of play will be an important part of the child's stay — the most important part of the day as far as he is concerned. Knowledge of the developmental needs of children will help those responsible to provide meaningful and acceptable play materials. As well as individual toys, the equipment can be made welcoming and less threatening by having equipment children recognise as being for them to use. The mere fact of being confined to bed need not preclude children from entering the great majority of play activities and, using a little imagination, life can become much more normal.

References

Barton, P.H. (1962). 'Play as a Tool of the Nurse', *Nursing Outlook,* 10, 162.

BBC (1975). *Toys,* London.

Boston Children's Medical Center (1969). *What to Do When There's Nothing to Do,* London: Hutchinson.

Harvey, S. and Hales-Tooke, A. (1972). *Play in Hospital,* London: Faber & Faber.

Jolly, H. (1968). 'Play and the Sick Child', *The Lancet,* 2, 1286.

MacCarthy, D. (1979). *The Under Fives in Hospital,* London: NAWCH.

Nash, S. (1976). *What is a Play Worker?*, NAWCH newsletter, summer 1976.

Newson, J. and E. (1979). *Toys and Playthings,* London: George Allen & Unwin.

Noble, E. (1967). *Play and the Sick Child,* London: Faber & Faber.

Petrillo, M. and Sanger, S. (1972). *The Emotional Care of the Hospitalised Child,* Philadelphia: Lippincott.

Plank, E. (1971). *Working with Children in Hospital,* Cleveland: Press of Case-Western Reserve, Second Edition.

Savage, J.H. (1975). 'A Cot Drawing Board', *The Nursing Times* 21 August 1975.

Savage, John H. (1977). 'Mattress Tilting Device', *The Nursing Mirror,* 2 June 1977.

Places Mentioned

Bellevue Hospital, New York.

Bramdean Hospital (school), Warwickshire.

Children's Hospital, Phoenix, Arizona.

General Hospital, Rugby.

James Whitcomb Riley Hospital, Indianapolis.

Liverpool Hospital for Children (country branch school).

Newhaven Hospital, Yale.

Stanford Children's Hospital, Palo Alto, California.

Stoke Mandeville Hospital, Aylesbury, Bucks.

University Hospital of Wales, Cardiff.

University Hospital, Denver, Colorado.

6 Communicating with Children

Introduction

It is just as erroneous to expect young children to understand adult concepts, as it is to say there is no use telling the child, as he won't understand anyway. Children are extremely sensitive to atmosphere. As adults, what we do may not be as important as what we say and how we behave. It is very necessary for us to understand how children think, if we are to establish meaningful relationships and adequately communicate with them.

Margaret Donaldson in her book *Children's Minds* (1978) states we may underestimate children's abilities to understand if we judge them by our adult concepts. Madeleine Petrillo in her book *The Emotional Care of the Hospitalised Child* (1972) describes many instances where, by using dolls and diagrams she was able to get through to quite young children concepts that could never be understood by language alone.

The establishment of communication with sick children is such a vital subject for us that separate sections are included on preparing children for a hospital visit, explaining medical and surgical procedures, as well as ways and means of speaking to children at a level they understand. Naturally, these will vary with age. A child's rate of development and understanding is influenced by various factors. Under stress, such as a hospitalisation, ability to understand may be impaired. On the other hand, any experience can be used positively if the child does not feel too threatened by it.

Children of all ages use play as an expression as well as a model on which to learn and come to terms with painful experiences. Painting, play-acting, dressing-up, active aggressive play, all can be used in this way. Children enjoy copying and love helping. Even in acute hospital wards these methods can be adopted. There are some ages when certain things assume greater importance than others. Armed with this sort of information, the nurse will find it much easier to help her young patient, especially if she also knows the special words each child uses for bowel actions, urination and the penis. Try checking these with mothers at the time of admission as well as the names of the rest of the family, including what they call their parents, food preferences and specially if they still take a bottle to bed. It is surprising how many quite big children enjoy this comfort. Whatever one's own views, a visit to hospital is not the time to break habits like this, or the use of a dummy — whatever the parents say. Even if the nursing process is not practised in the unit as a whole, write it on a separate card and pin it to the end of the child's cot, so all can see and use it.

Because there are specific needs at certain ages I have re-iterated those that have particular significance for communication (see Chapter 4).

Different Age Groups

THE UNDER THREES

Even children under two may understand simple explanations, but often cannot retain them. They should be in visual terms and repeated. As the children are too emotionally immature to relate to a series of adults, their ability to understand what a mother says may be much greater than if the same thing is conveyed to them by a stranger. It is also quite difficult for other adults to understand what young children are saying, although this may be quite clear to the mother. Explanations should then be given in the presence of the parent and reinforced by them. For example, a dressing procedure can be demonstrated by bandaging a teddy bear.

Explaining that 'Mummy' will come tomorrow is a concept a child of this age just cannot comprehend. It may be possible to convey if it is linked with a definite and recognised time such as 'after breakfast'. As any separation at this age is likely

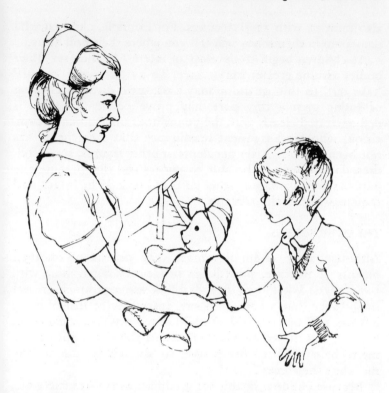

to be regarded as an abandonment, it will help the child to retain an image of Mummy if she is asked to leave some tangible evidence of herself, such as a glove or handbag. For older children a photograph to keep on the locker will provide a focus so nurses and other staff can talk with the child about his family.

THE FOUR TO SIX YEAR OLDS

Children of this age have a vivid imagination and often are thrilled by the magical. Fantasy may play a large part in their games of make-believe. Some develop imaginary playmates, who are so real that adults can hold quite serious conversations with them. Even when the child finds it impossible to describe what is troubling him, be it pain, fear or anger, he is able to tell you through the imaginary friend. Dolls and teddies are also imbued with these feelings. For example, children who deny pain in themselves will tell you where their doll hurts.

As children begin to develop an interest in their sex, their bodies assume greater importance. To use the word 'cut off' 'take out' to this age group may cause great distress. The fear of losing even a tiny part may prove devastating. This is demonstrated clearly with the young boys undergoing circumcision, who need frequent reassurance that their 'penis' has not been cut off. After accidents or other trauma, some children do not seem to be able to understand that because one part has been damaged, other parts of him may be intact, and they may need help over this.

THE OVER SEVENS

Although some children remain very dependent on their parents at this age, most begin to identify much more with their peers. What their friends think assumes much greater importance than what adults say. Insecurity or fear of being left can still be very real. A child of ten was distraught when her bed was moved to another part of the ward. She begged me to be sure to tell her mother so 'she will be able to find me when she comes'.

Because children in this age group are active and energetic, great sensitivity will be needed towards the bed-bound child who, apart from an orthopaedic condition, is feeling well. His level of frustration may prove impossible for him to handle without help.

ADOLESCENTS

The emotional turmoil of the adolescent makes him difficult to help; he may want just as much caring for as a young child at the same time as the rights and privileges of the adult world. Young people of this age become re-aware of themselves and their emerging physical maturity. They may be preoccupied and suffer acutely from fears of the future but find it hard to talk about unless they are very sure of the adult's interest and support. Adolescents are particularly sensitive to criticism and can be acutely embarrassed at remarks that a year or so earlier they would have shrugged off.

Ways to Communicate

All learning is reckoned to be incomplete if it relies on the spoken word only. It may be enhanced by visual aids, but participation is needed if full understanding is to be gained. This rule needs to be followed closely with children. Just telling will never suffice. Words can have very different meanings for children, who may understand something very different from what the adult meant to convey. As words are so misleading, they must be chosen with care. 'Will you?' and 'May I?' are dangerous if you are looking for cooperation. Avoid such words as 'take out' or 'cut off' and try replacing them with less threatening words such as that the doctor will 'fix it', 'mend it' or 'repair it'. These will convey the meaning quite satisfactorily without frightening the child into horrors of mutilation.

Children in hospital will be home-sick and probably unhappy at times. This is understandable. The nurse will try to comfort or divert the child's attention, but if she is unable to do so, may well blame herself and abandon the scene, leaving the child to sob himself to sleep. Although, sadly, unhappiness is at times an inevitable part of a hospital experience, it is not necessary to leave a child comfortless. Some wards use the baby slings now in use by many mothers, which allows one to continue using both hands whilst the baby remains in close cuddling contact. Ordinary push-chairs or small prams can be used in the ward to allow the child to stay close. They also feel more at home than rolling around in a large open cot. Some units have adapted the prams so that drip poles can be inserted. A cuddle and a listening ear will do wonders.

As children get older they sometimes feel they shouldn't cry and try terribly hard not to. I have found occasionally that one has to show it does not matter if they do cry and you will understand. Gently talking about Mummy, home, admitting you know how he would like to be with them, can be comforting, if at the same time you are cuddling and perhaps gently rocking him. Even if the child begins to cry it isn't always wise to stop him until he has been able to 'get it out of his system'. It may be easier and less traumatic for the nurse to cheer him up, but it may drive the pain and anguish of the child inwards.

Children see a great deal more than adults suppose. It can never be assumed they have not heard and seen everything that is going on in the ward. It needs to be rememberd that, although they may have seen and heard, the conclusions they come to about these things may be very different from the way adults view them.

Jackie, a 4 year old who had a permanent tracheotomy, greeted me when I came on duty one morning with 'Sister, did you know a baby died in there last night?', pointing to the bathroom. 'Yes', I replied, wondering what she would say next. 'Did they kill it in there?', she then asked. 'No one killed the baby, Jackie — the baby died because he wasn't strong enough to breathe anymore.' Jackie thought for a moment and then added 'I was like that once wasn't I, but I was too strong.'

Not only had the staff assured me that everyone had been asleep, but had I been too quick with my answer we might not have known Jackie really thought the baby had been killed. What might the implications of that sort of memory be?

Lynne was being taken to theatre when loud screams were heard coming from the adjacent recovery room. She had been well premedicated and was lying apparently asleep. I kept looking at her. Did she hear the child's screams? If she did, did it worry her? Should I point it out so I could explain — but if I did and the child hadn't heard or been worried, would it not in fact have made it worse for her? Finally, I decided that she must have heard. 'Do you hear that child crying, Lynne?' I ventured, 'Yes', she breathed, opening her eyes which I then saw were very troubled. I was able to explain 'That's Diane. She's had her tonsils out and wants to go back to the ward.' Lynne visibly sank back into the hard theatre trolley. I had been unaware of how rigid and tense she had been before.

If we are to improve our techniques in talking with children and helping them with their feelings and experiences in hospital, there are no short cuts. We will need to be constantly on the alert, using all our skill in sensitive observation and be prepared to wait for and listen to what the children tell us. Without this we cannot hope to really communicate meaningfully.

Preparing Children for Hospital

Hospital is not an isolated experience affecting only a few unfortunate children. A quarter of the British child population will spend at least one night in hospital before they are seven. In addition to this, many more will find their way to accident and emergency departments for cuts, fractures, sutures. Because the vast majority of children are admitted as emergencies, whether for accidents or medical conditions, it is not feasible to suggest that adequate preparation can be done once admission is agreed. A few hospitals are experimenting with video-tapes and slides depicting scenes of ward life that the child can be shown while he is waiting admission in casualty. Many more produce their own leaflets giving information about facilities, regulations and things the patient should bring. Neither of these will ever be able adequately to prepare him for the shock of coming into hospital suddenly. It is, however, very possible to include information about hospitals in education. Television programmes have made certain parts familiar. As it affects so many younger children, play groups, nursery and infant schools will be good places to begin. Voluntary agencies such as NAWCH (National Association for the Welfare of Children in Hospital) help by showing slides and giving illustrated talks about hospital, but nothing will be so welcome as a real live nurse — in uniform of course!

Arranging for groups of children to be taken round the children's wards, showing them things that as patients they would be bound to see can be a positive learning experience. For example, many children do not know hospital beds have wheels, 'so you can be pushed in them'. Point out the ward with lots of beds in it — the bedside locker, the bed table to eat or play on, the unfamiliar bedpan or bottle, curtains that pull round the beds instead of doors and walls, and, of course, the nurses. Children are often surprised that a 'nurse stays awake all night just in case you want her'. To know there is television, a play-room, even school, what the toilets and bathrooms look like, all can be reassuring to the child.

When children know they are to be admitted, it is good to be able to invite them up to the ward beforehand. Some hospitals run a puppet show to familiarise the prospective patients with the routine of hospital life. A story illustrated by pictures, slides and one or two actual hospital items such as a mask, name bracelet, bottle or bedpan, brings the scenes to life. Sending out a special invitation to the child to visit at the same time as the hospital informs the parents of admission can make the child feel welcomed. We used to send out a duplicated leaflet saying:

> The doctor has said you need to come into hospital.
> We should like you to visit us in the children's ward beforehand, so you know what it will be like.
> We expect you want to know all sorts of things:
>> Where you will sleep?
>> What you do all day?
>> Where you keep your things?
>> Where you eat?
>> Even where you have operations?
> We can show you. You can meet the people who look after you in hospital.
> Why don't you bring Mummy (and Daddy if he can come) to . . . . . . ward at . . . . . . when we can show you round.
> You can invite your brother or sister to come as well if you like.
> SEE YOU FRIDAY

Some larger units and children's hospitals may be able to organise conducted tours. In one place I visited in the United States a pre-admission party is arranged every fortnight. Medical and nursing staff and students combine to put on a mime depicting a child being admitted to hospital — greeted by the receptionist, put into a cot and then exmained. A meal is then brought for the child to eat in bed. Later the parents say good-night and go home. A narrator tells the story. It is simply acted but very effective. Afterwards children have a chance of playing with hospital equipment which has been laid out ready. I saw a doctor instructing a child how to look down his throat and others dressing up in outsize gowns, masks and gloves.

There are a number of excellent books on the market today to read to children about hospital and most children's libraries stock some of them. The National Association for the Welfare of Children in Hospital (NAWCH) provide a selection of these if they are difficult to obtain locally. It is a good idea if the hospital shop or league of friends can stock the cheaper ones. They may take them, too, on their trolleys if they go round the out-patient departments.

Many hospitals now have their own admission leaflets which describe briefly the facilities that can be expected, but rarely give enough information for the children to know what it is actually like to be a patient. It can be useful to contact the local health clinics, GP surgeries and health visitors. They are good sources, both for the supply and dissemination of information to families of young children.

With the cooperation of health education departments and the community medical and nursing services, it is possible to do a great deal to educate the young family in case of need. As over 85% of medical admissions may be emergencies (according to one survey in 1976) this sort of preparation is bound to be of great value. Health visitors have the advantage of knowing the family circumstances and will also be able to support the family after the child is discharged, often a time when the family feels badly neglected. Many units now have liaison health visitors who can be invaluable links, both to parents and staff (see Chapter 9).

Just because some children may have been to see a hospital before, or even accepted an invitation to visit the ward prior to admission, there can be no guarantee that they will have remembered details. Alternatively, details they did see may have been erroneously interpreted or remembered as the 'main thing' in hospital.

Children need simple explanations of what they see when they are admitted. It is well worth time spent looking at the ward from the child's eye view. Watch what they stare at — ask them what they think it is and then correct them as necessary. Simple words and explanations are the only ones

they will retain so it may be necessary to start re-training ourselves to speak in ordinary lay language and everyday terms.
The oxygen tent is easily described as the little house (or tent)
with specially good air for breathing; the incubator — a type
of space ship, or greenhouse perhaps — which is kept so nice
and warm the baby doesn't need clothes on; the sucker — the
machine that helps people cough when they find it difficult.
Children are often worried when they see a naso-gastric tube,
intravenous fluids, gallows traction and some other orthopaedic equipment.

Preparing Children for Treatment

This section is directed mainly at the school-age child. For
the child under four the important thing is to prepare the
parent, as the child will be unlikely to retain much of what
he is told.

BLOOD TESTS

Once children are admitted, they will be subjected to many
new and baffling experiences. Even the taking of blood may
cause confusion. Children have been known to describe the
phlebotomist as a 'vampire' or 'blood sucker', a term understood when one watches them using a pipette to draw blood.
Another child was overheard to say 'They stuck a needle in
and stole my blood; they don't want me to have any!'

> Martin, aged 14, who was in the last stages of leukaemia
> became upset at the frequency of blood tests. 'I am very
> worried — they are taking too much blood. I know I don't
> have enough.' What he did not say was that by taking all
> his blood he would die. This needed to be discussed, but in
> order to show him the relative insignificance of 20 mls
> blood I used two large jugs of water to approximate to his
> blood volume. He then chose the biggest syringe and re-
> moved some water from one of the jugs. He squirted it
> into a small glass. It helped to see how little blood had
> really been taken. This then gave us a chance to talk about
> the real issue.

Before starting on any campaign of preparation, it is imperative that one tells the child the truth. It is pointless to say something won't hurt when it obviously will. One child commented 'They said it wouldn't hurt — only because it doesn't hurt them. They don't know how it feels.' Many of us say these things because, frankly, we hope it won't hurt. We dislike the idea of inflicting pain and tend to deny its existence. It is much better to say 'I know it will hurt, but only for a minute. You can shout if you like!' Telling a child 'to be brave' may make it harder to bear.

PRE-OPERATIVE CARE

Whether the preparation is for a test, examination or a major procedure such as an operation, or applying a plaster cast, it is important to get the timing right. Start preparation for something major in good time to allow the child to get used to it. Talking round the subject, stories, games, all will help to familiarise the child and need not provoke anxiety if given in a straightforward way. Do not dwell on details or on any procedure that the child will not be conscious of. Children are far more interested in the fact that they may miss breakfast, or have a special gown 'split down the back' to wear, than the details of checking premedications, or identification bracelets. To let children have a ride on the theatre trolley, see a nurse dress up in theatre clothing, and then experiment themselves, means that operation day need have no surprises for them. It is important that children believe what is told them, but equally important that what they believe is what they actually experience. Try asking children to report back afterwards, to make sure you have told them the truth. It may surprise you what children remember and say. One quite mature girl, who had had a previously traumatic anaesthetic, which she vividly described, told me afterwards that 'everything you told me was true except for one thing — I didn't have an operation!' She thought about this for a moment and then said, 'I suppose I must have done.'

When explanations have to be given, try using everyday language. This will make it much more intelligible to your patient. I always try to explain the reason for insulin to a diabetic, for example, by describing a pair of scales. As the body has stopped making its own insulin we have to provide it. Because we aren't as clever as our bodies, who know just the right amount we need, we have to balance the insulin according to what we eat. This is the reason we need to eat the same sort of amounts of food each day to keep well. In a similar way pyloric stenosis can be described to parents as a tight rubber band round the outlet pipe from the stomach; kidneys, the sieves that separate the water from the food in your bloodstream; haematuria — when the holes in the sieve get too big; and the bladder, like a balloon that stretches to hold the urine or 'wee'. There will be many ways of explaining but 'The doctor knows how to make it better' is a good standby.

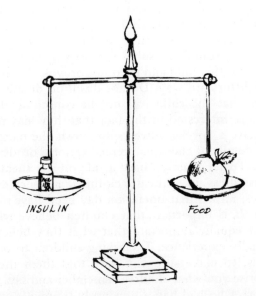

Children need to be given the simple facts in language they can understand. By asking a child prior to a tonsillectomy where his tonsils are and how the doctor is going to remove them, all sorts of misconceptions are corrected. One child of six I nursed had been told by his mother that the doctor would take them out with a special sort of spoon — near enough to an accurate description for me to use in future preparing of children. This child was also told the doctor would give him a 'magic sleep' first, which he obviously thought would be fun.

Don't forget some children may find the whole prospect too unbearable to be able to talk about. By talking to a small group of children who say they want to know, the more anxious one can listen without becoming too involved. If such a child persists with a high level of anxiety, it is probably wise to postpone the procedure, or operation, until he has come to terms with the stress. Of course, this is not always possible. One young boy of seven with an unstable fracture, who had been transferred to us from an adult ward, was acutely anxious. Unfortunately, having waited all day to go

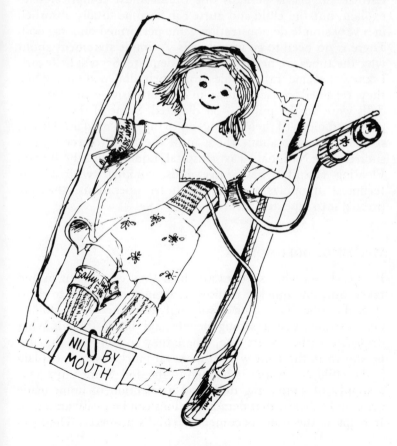

to the theatre, he was finally called in a hurry and there was no time for adequate premedication. By making sure he was accompanied by a senior nurse, whom he trusted and who had in fact prepared him, he was anaesthetised without distress. During the afternoon the nurse had showed him some plaster of Paris and then let him soak it and put it on a doll's leg. He watched it get hard and talked about how it would come off. He soon considered himself the ward expert on his own plaster cast!

CARDIAC SURGERY

Cardiac surgery is perhaps one of the most complicated to explain, but the child and nurse can become totally absorbed in a very simple demonstration game performed on a rag doll. There is no need to go into details. A simple statement about why the tubes are needed is quite adequate. Several little girls I knew became inseparable from their doll patients. When they regained consciousness in the intensive-care unit, the dolls were on the pillow — as directed. Some of the children projected much of their feelings on to the doll 'models'. Others seemingly forgot about them until the time for removal of sutures. The National Heart Hospital, London and the Boston Floating Hospital, have large dolls, complete with all the technical trappings needed for heart operations, that are pressed into repeated use.

THE USE OF DOLL MODELS

If one shows what stitches are, how they can be put in and taken out, one quickly realises how much easier it is to show than describe. Try using a soft polyurethane or rag doll to demonstrate. Use a strong needle and black thread. What drips and catheters are like, where they go and why, can also be shown in the same way. It makes it much easier to explain if the child can watch it happen to the doll. Some units have a supply of simple rag dolls and a selection of home-made drips and tubes so that demonstrations can be easily arranged. It helps if the dolls become the child's property. They can then be used to 'play out' some of the hospital experiences. With some children this goes on for weeks or months.

BURNS AND SCALDS

In a burns unit at the Riley Children's Hospital, Indianapolis, rag dolls are used in the same sort of way. Each child on admission receives a doll and is encouraged to cut out the area on the doll that 'hurts'. Invariably the child cuts out the area approximating to his burn. All except once, as was explained to me, when the child cut out a large area on the doll's back, although her only apparent injury was in a totally different place. When asked why, she said 'because that's where it hurts'. The head nurse probed: 'Is that where you hurt too?' 'Yes', came the reply. There had been no indication or complaint to suggest the child was at all uncomfortable on her back. This discomfort was relieved at once. The dolls in this unit accompany the patients to all their treatments including baths. After grafting, a piece of gauze is sewn (by the child) on the affected place. Before discharge, the original piece that had been removed is sewn back by the child of course. Some of the dolls become regular out-patients with their owners.

HELPING THE UNDER THREES

When children are very tiny, it is even more difficult to know how to communicate as their vocabulary is restricted and understanding limited. Having felt impotent to help a 20-month-old severely scalded child, whose hands and feet were hidden by huge occlusive bandages, it was a relief to learn that in fact one could easily show even such a tiny child that underneath those monstrous gloves her hands and feet were still there. By using a precious teddy, taking his paws and bandaging them and unwrapping them over and over again, one could repeat 'See teddy's hand, see teddy's foot is still there.'

This particular child went through agonies. One could see the child was totally bewildered. She had returned from the operating theatre with bulky fist bandages which she could in no way use as hands. She gradually lapsed into a depressed withdrawal. Despite everyone's efforts to rouse or interest her, it was not until some weeks later when the bandages were removed that she showed any liveliness again. If only we had known in time how to get through to her. I shall always be grateful to Madeleine Petrillo for her research and sensitivity in this area of nursing.

Explaining Tests

The same methods can be used for children with frog plasters and insertion of spitz-holder valves and they can be used to show many of the investigations children undergo. Electro-encephalogram leads, catheters, naso-gastric tubes, prostheses of all descriptions can be demonstrated and explained so much more easily on a model. In many hospitals, experienced play staff participate in the delicate task of explaining beforehand and then helping the child afterwards to understand what has happened to him (see Chapter 9).

THE WARD MASCOT

Another hospital uses an outsize monkey similar to 'Zozo' of the hospital-book fame. He is the ward mascot and accompanies the nurse preparing every new child for his treatment. All the equipment a child is likely to actually see for his particular treatment is kept in a labelled box. The appropriate set is put on the child's bed complete with 'Zozo' the monkey, who is to have the same operation as the patient. On a pretext the nurse leaves the child alone to investigate the box and usually by the time she returns it is already well explored. One of the items in the box is always a medi-swab, as children are often surprised by its coldness and smell.

OTHER USEFUL AIDS

Outline diagrams of the body are also most useful to help explanations. They can be used successfully for parents too, by medical staff. These were pioneered by Emma Plank (1962), who also used dolls extensively. Books and pictures

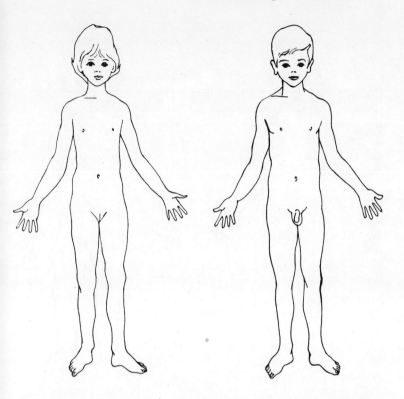

may also be used. One child-life worker in Cleveland made a
'preparation for operation' book which was used to augment
the verbal explanations. It had a three-dimensional aspect.
Little flaps over the masked faces of the attendants, nurses
and doctors, when lifted, revealed their normal smiling faces.
Similarly the sheet could be lifted off the theatre trolley. You
could see children found it reassuring to discover the patient
was still whole. When children can do so it sometimes helps
to allow them to actually assist in the procedure. One ten
year old I knew was extremely fearful of having sutures removed after surgery for aortic stenosis. He became totally
absorbed when under careful tutelage he removed all the
stitches himself. His technique was totally aseptic. A potentially hazardous procedure with an hysterical child was
turned into one of triumph for the patient and relief for
the nurse!

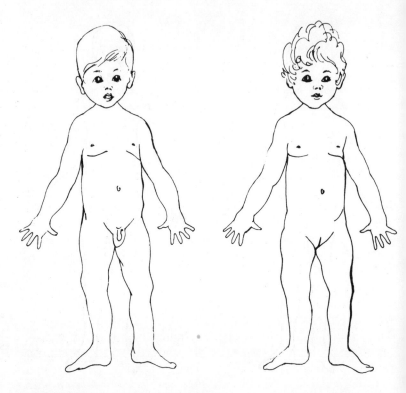

Communicating with the Family

Communication with children is one of the great delights of paediatrics, especially when it is seen to help overcome fears, stresses, and the sometimes almost insuperable problems facing the sick child. But it can never be truly regarded as wholly satisfactory unless communication includes the parents — indeed the whole family.

It is a sad fact that much of what children hear from their parents about illness is a reflection of the parent's own understanding and that may be coloured by their own unhappy experiences. They may need more help than the child, particularly if the child is likely to have a permanent handicap of some sort. Verbal communication alone is never enough. The involvement of the child by watching and even practising is required, but of equal importance is the skill of listening to what the child has to tell us.

LISTENING

Dr MacCarthy (1974) reflected that it is not easy to have the patience to listen to children. We often find it so much easier to fill in the gaps, or finish the sentence for them. Asking questions that have a 'Yes' or 'No' answer will be good conversation-stoppers and reveal nothing about the way the child feels. When a child asks a question, try turning it round and ask the same thing back to the child or reply in a questioning tone 'That's how you feel about it, is it?'

Although children may misunderstand what an adult says, they certainly will view the problem from their own inimitable standpoint. Children are almost always ready to communicate with an adult they trust. They quickly ferret out those who really care enough to listen long enough. They also need someone who will respect them enough to tell them the truth. It is essential not to laugh, dismiss or underestimate what is said, and be able to keep a confidence when asked to do so.

Many children feel they have to put on a brave face to their parents, and they also try hard to be brave in hospital. The strain of this can be overwhelming and the relief at finding someone with whom it is safe to be sad, to cry, to express doubts and fears cannot be over-emphasised.

Children also need the adults to know how to cope with any given situation. Nothing throws children quicker than indecision. On the other hand, they will respect you if you say you do not know the answer but that you will try to find out.

Summary

Despite our dedication to the total care of sick children and concern to keep the family intact, it must be admitted there are many imperfections in our communication with them. So often we are surprised at the way they react; we need to prepare them every step of the way. We have to recognise that children feel isolated when they are in hospital. They regard it as being planned by and for adults who are too busy to be bothered with them, thus they remain aliens in an adult world. If they are to feel they matter we need to communicate at a level they understand. To do so we must employ the tools they use and the language they speak. We will have to put ourselves in their place.

Nothing can take the place of human contact. Each sick child is an individual and has the right to be treated with respect as such. We must rise to the challenge to get alongside each young patient and his parents as they struggle with hospital and sickness, to learn how they think and feel; to help them understand. We owe it to them to tell the truth, but we also need the ability and determination to always interpret that truth in love.

References

Donaldson, M. (1978). *Children's Minds,* London: Fontana/ Collins.

Macarthy, D. (1974). 'Communication between Children and Doctors', *Developmental Medicine and Child Neurology,* 16, 3, 279–285.

Lowenstein, H. (1979). 'Some "Funny Things" Happened on the Way to the Theatre', *The Nursery World,* 5 July 1979.

Petrillo, M. and Sanger, S. (1972). *The Emotional Care of the Hospitalised Child,* Philadelphia: Lippincott.

Plank, E. (1962). *Working with Children in Hospital,* Cleveland: Press of Case-Western Reserve. Second edition 1971.

Special Books for Children

Althea Books (1974). *Going to the Doctor,* Dinosaur.

Althea Books (1974). *Going to the Hospital,* Dinosaur.

Jessel, C. (1972). *Paul in Hospital,* London: Methuen.

Jessel, C. (1975). *Mark's Wheelchair Adventures,* London: Methuen.

Peacock, F. (1976). *The Hospital,* Franklin Watts.

Rey, M. and H. (1967). *Zozo Goes to Hospital* (*Curious George*), Chatto & Windus.

Simpson, J. (1973). *Come and See the Hospital,* Felix Gluck.

Preparation for Death of Relative/Friend

Buchanan-Smith, D. (1975). *A Taste of Blackberries*, London: Heinemann.
Fassler, J. (1971). *My Grandpa Died Today*, Human Sciences Press.
Fassler, J. (1971). *The Boy with a Problem*, Behaviour Publications.

Places Mentioned

Boston Children's Medical Center.
Boston Floating Hospital.
Charing Cross Hospital, Fulham.
Cornell Medical Center, New York.
James Whitcomb Riley Hospital, Indianapolis.
National Heart Hospital, London.
Rainbow Babies Hospital, Cleveland.
Washington Children's Hospital, Washington, D.C.

7 Creating the Right Environment

Introduction

When Lorraine, aged 13, said of hospital 'It's like being lonesome all the time', she was not speaking of physical isolation. In a recent survey undertaken for the Consumer Association (1980) practically all the children interviewed expressed the same sort of thing. In hospital they felt isolated, with no one who really had time to know what they thought, what they wanted, how they felt. It was all right for people like Mum: 'It was nice in her ward but it wasn't where I was.'

First Impressions

A great deal is being done in hospitals today to make them more attractive — plants, easy chairs, pictures, carpeting. But often the only indication that an area is designated for children is a table with chipped paint and small chairs. Tattered comics and a box of ill-assorted toys make up the decor. This isn't true of most children's wards. But many children are nursed in adult wards or in side rooms or bays, particularly in specialist disciplines. Accident and emergency departments rarely have room to create a special children's waiting area, away from the main stream of casualties and emergency admissions. Yet it is now strongly recommended by the British Paediatric Association that all children coming to accident and emergency departments should be received in a separate area.

Guys-Evelina Hospital London is one of the very few general hospitals in this country that run a separate children's casualty. Even this hospital cannot maintain a 24-hour service. Children are received in the main department at night and at weekends.

Yet children make up the majority of patients seen in many accident and emergency departments and it is frequently their first introduction to hospital life. What happens and what is seen colour future impressions. Apart from road-traffic accidents, many children are brought up to the accident and emergency departments by-passing their general practitioners.

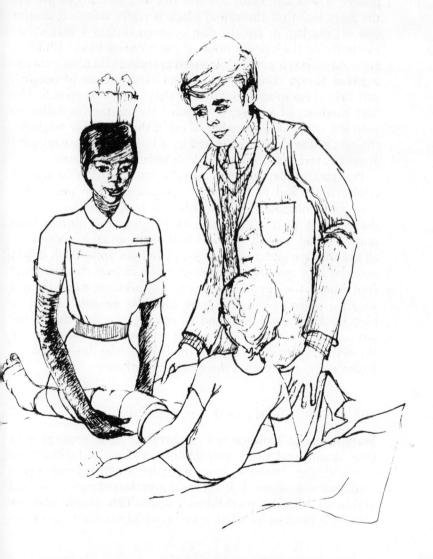

Departments

X-ray departments and fracture clinics treat a large number of children too. They can be most forbidding places and are almost always adult-orientated. Mobiles, posters, and using toys to attract attention rather than snapping of fingers are always worthwhile. A short time spent explaining that the plaster is wet and cold, but will dry and go hard to protect the hurt leg, that the round blade is really safe – it cannot saw off the leg, or cut the skin as seems certain – may offset the terror of the hideous noise of the whirring blade. Children are used to staying still while snaps are being taken, so explaining that X-rays take 'special photos of the inside of people', will help them to understand that they have to keep still. The best method, of course, is to have the mother or father in with the child. Do remember to ask if the mother is pregnant, though, so she can be protected by a lead apron. One hospital always covers these aprons with flowery cotton prints.

Out-patient departments usually have to double up for adult clinics and in specialist units the children and adults may have combined clinics. This may be little different from the familiar doctor's surgery, except that the waiting time may be much longer. Mothers will most probably arrive with all the children under school age in tow, and apart from drinks and the loo, may need somewhere to change the baby and feed him if the appointment is at an awkward time. Do not forget a place to put the pram safely is essential. Ideally a play worker should be found to run a play group during the out-patient clinics. In this case the children stop complaining, the mother stops worrying and the baby settles down to sleep. Without any occupation there can be bedlam.

THE ADVANTAGE OF STAFF WHO LIKE CHILDREN

Staff who like children will be invaluable, as tempers wear thin at the end of a busy children's clinic if facilities are cramped and diversion for the patients and accompanying siblings non-existent. It helps for out-patient clinics to be held within or adjacent to children's units. This means that the staff will become familiar both to children about to be admitted and those attending for follow-up clinics. Specialist clinics as those described for diabetic patients (Chapter 4) can sometimes be run by the same team responsible for the in-patients. When children are to be admitted from the clinic it is good to let them see the ward and meet the people beforehand. It is also good if all blood tests can be done at this time, too. An experienced technician or doctor will make all the difference to the child's attitude if other tests are needed later.

At one hospital where I worked there was a technician who loved working with the children. She never minded taking time to gain the child's co-operation first and asked that the children should all be sent for at a certain time so she could be sure of having time to spend with them. Most of them came out with minute faces drawn on plastered finger tips with biro or little snow caps of cotton wool.

There are other departments, too, in hospitals, which children and adults attend together. The electro-encephalogram department is one area where young children are frequently sent but which can prove very traumatic. Although it is difficult to get these young children to cooperate alone, there are still many departments who do not welcome parents with their young children. Once they can be persuaded to, however, they almost always become advocates of the idea, especially if child and parents have been well prepared beforehand about what to expect. Having a large doll on which to demonstrate helps to explain to parents as well as their children what is required. A series of photos taken of children during the test are sometimes used to augment verbal explanation. The anaesthetic room and theatre reception area can also be made more amenable to child patients. Pictures on the ceilings and mobiles help, but please look critically at the areas where children in your hospital may go to try to see things the way they may see them. Some children are fascinated by the 'tools they do operations with'; others are sure they are used only for the grossest mutilations.

The Wards

Most children's wards have been adapted from the general ward plan laid down for the whole hospital; a few lucky ones have had units tailor-made for their needs. Even in new hospitals children are expected to fit in with the multi-purpose design of the ward block. The unit that has managed to get a ground floor site, access to a roof-garden area or outdoor play space, is indeed fortunate. It is certain that administrators will need to be convinced that paediatric needs are really different and that these differences are justified. What then are the priorities for a children's ward?

SAFETY

Children can be like quicksilver when they want to get some-where. Not only are they incredibly quick, but they may be unbelievably young! Windows, doors, particularly the swing door type, must be made safe. Staircases and lifts must be child-proof and away from their reach. It is surprising how often this is not so. One unit I worked in was very proud of its new laundry shoot. Delightfully easy to use, it was large enough to take a full linen skip without any difficulty. It was conveniently sited well away from observation. But there were no means of securing the door. My imagination soared – what a wonderful place to hide – or even better, to push unsuspecting Danny or even nurse! It might have fatal con-sequences. Low cupboards for lotions, medicines, testing equipment, cleaning materials too, must all be kept locked. Many two or three year olds land up in hospital because of overdoses of the most bizarre solutions. One Christmas, we admitted two very inebriated little boys. The parents were not amused as they had drunk all the Christmas liquor. Another time we were entranced by the pervading scent of Chanel No. 5. Mother, whose precious present it had been, found it hard to be glad her child was none the worse for her illicit drink. One can never assume children are discerning over what is safe. Unprotected radiators, electric-socket out-lets at convenient bedhead height, toilets lockable only from inside and inaccessible from without, thermometer holders, windows, staircases – all pose hazards in the paediatric wards. It is not only new units that have dangers; oxygen cylinders left standing without carriers can be a constant headache to staff.

Hydraulic beds have been decreed unsafe for children's wards because of the danger that a young child may become trapped in the mechanism, which is capable of crunching a skull without so much as a hiccough. Yet many wards where children are nursed are using them. The manually operated variable-height beds present no such danger and have the added attraction of being cheaper. Fixed-height beds are very difficult for younger children to get on and off. They seem adept at falling off them, but hate the indignity of cot-sides. Cots have their snags too. Older children (over threes who normally at home sleep in low divans or bunk beds) may be put into cots purely for safety. Many object strongly to bars. They climb over, walk along the rails, lean over and undo the cot sides. Harnesses and restrainers are officially discouraged and should only be used with the written permission of the consultant in charge. Children with head injuries who are restless and disorientated must be protected. It is possible to nurse very restless ones on mattresses on the floor, or even in a playpen. Older children will settle sometimes on one of the parents' bed-chairs, if they are low and semi-protected. Adaptations have been made to cots and one we found totally satisfactory for cots was made by a volunteer. Fitted on the ends of the cot it effectively raised the height of the sides without restricting access to the child or making it like a 'cage'. When not in use it could be folded back to make a trough for toys above the cot or removed altogether.

ATMOSPHERE

The atmosphere of a ward does not depend on the opulence of its furnishings, or the extent of its facilities. It depends on the attitudes of the staff. Where these are really child- and family-centred their needs are understood and met. Some of these needs will centre round the arrangements made for the parent's comfort, others around the desires for families to continue their life-style as far as possible. One of the most comforting and reassuring things in a ward is to be able to see the person looking after you. When the nurses' station or sister's office is out of sight, not only does it hinder the professional's observation but it can seriously undermine the security of the patient. More than this, it reinforces the distance between patient and staff, and parent and staff. When there is no such barrier the sister's desk is not only the hub of the wheel but it becomes a 'honey-pot' to the children. Occasionally one might wish for a respite but this is a small price to pay.

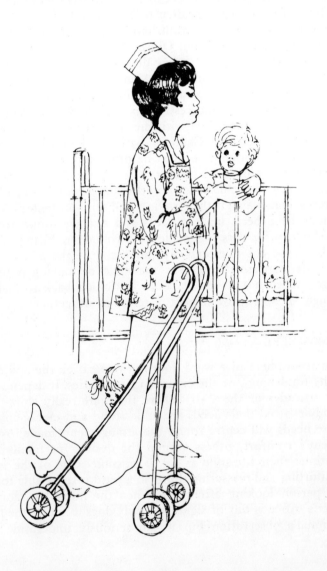

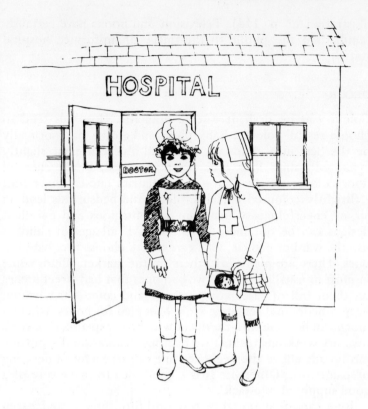

UNIFORM

The insecurity and bewilderment that patients and relatives feel when exposed to the rather formidable hospital image, can be minimised by informality. Wearing of coloured smocks or overalls over the new white nurses' uniforms immediately dispels some of the distance they create between staff and patient. In some units uniform has been dispensed with altogether; in at least one all staff wear Laura Ashley print dresses. Certainly play staff and nursery nurses are often acceptable in mufti but, in the majority of hospitals, administrators are not willing to make exceptions to uniform for the paediatric staff. Doctors and paramedical staff will sometimes take off white coats, but then male nurses get the title instead. Obtaining authentic uniforms from the sewing room for the children to dress up in helps to lessen the gap (see illustration on p. 115). Television and books have certainly familiarised the public to the image of uniformed hospital staff.

DECOR

Colour can be drab, it can be dramatic. Hospitals tend to choose restful colours. Baby pinks and greens may not really be the best in a children's ward and blue can make slightly cyanosed babies look even more cyanosed. Bright cheerful door colours can be fun — in paediatrics one can have fun!

Brightly coloured curtains, blinds and bedspreads lend an air of cheerfulness which can be contagious and excellent designs can be obtained for children. If all ages of children use the ward or cubicle, take care not to choose too 'babyish' ones. There are plenty of others on the market. Blinds come in most unusual patterns — we had ones that had street scenes on them full of fascinating activity and colours that would keep a bedbound lethargic child occupied for hours. Whereas much can be done with the decor with little expense, children's own art work creates its own exciting decoration. By putting pin boards above the bedheads one can save a lot of defacing of paintwork. Otherwise it is a good idea to make sure of a good supply of 'blu-tack'.

By a careful appraisal of the ward furniture, it can be seen just how many 'strange-looking' items abound. Some cannot be avoided. Oxygen tents, suckers, tractions, incubators may well be in use. Examination trolleys, intravenous poles, medical and other supplies do not usually need to be left around. Some hospitals I know have decorated the medicine trolleys with transfers and make a point of explaining whatever equipment is in use to all new patients. When children need to have special tests, or specimens collected, it isn't always safe to expect them to remind the adults what is to be done or what they may or may not eat. Nil by Mouth signs I think are better described as 'Nothing to eat or drink'. This is much more intelligible to parents who, after all, may well be the custodians and caretakers. We found in one hospital that ordinary cardboard labels, with safety pins on the back, made good badges identifying those on diets, to have operations or

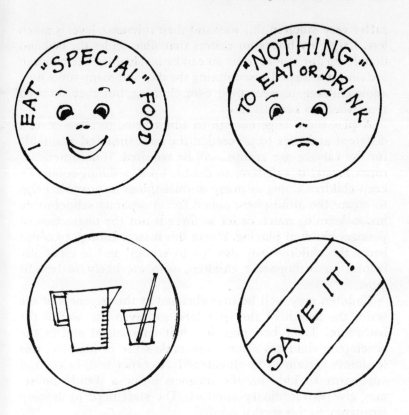

who needed fluids to be measured and collected. Children of all ages love badges. So this seems a satisfactory answer to problems when children are mobile, in and out of the playroom, schoolroom and ward areas. Children can also have fun making them if the designs are simple.

LIVING QUARTERS

First impressions are always important. In Chapter 5 it was pointed out that a large rocking horse gave a welcome and also a 'safe place' for the patient to view the ward. Children need plenty of space for their own belongings too. It is not hard to remember the frustration of having all your toys tossed unceremoniously into a box or cupboard. Some small precious items were never recovered. Children in hospital suffer very much in this way and their tolerance level is much less. Large toy boxes on casters that slide under the bed and double up for stools to sit on can be invaluable. The children are almost always dressed during the day and many units now allow children to wear their own clothing, but they do need somewhere to keep them.

A play-room large enough to admit beds, to allow several different activities to proceed at the same time and adaptable for the varying age groups, will be required. If no other day-room exists, it will have to double up as a dining-room. To keep children doing as many normal things as possible helps to create the atmosphere aimed for. A separate school-room makes learning much easier as there is not the distraction of younger children playing. Where this is large enough to admit beds, the children can also 'go to school' and is especially helpful to orthopaedic children, who are likely to benefit most.

Children may well be overwhelmed at the largeness of the ward, the length of the corridors, and even the size of the bathroom. Their bed may be their only island and as the developing child has a very vulnerable sense of identity, this is almost certain to be threatened. A corner bed, boxes and cupboards to hide in, the snugness inside a Wendy house, may give extraordinary comfort. The staff need to develop sensitivity to this sort of need.

RELATIONSHIPS

To a great extent, the atmosphere will depend on the relationships staff develop with the families. A few nurses still covet the satisfaction of taking a mother's place when the child is brought in as a patient. More sincerely believe they are the experts on child care and know best. Neither attitude will help the establishment of the partnership and mutual dedication to the care of the sick child. When the staff are truly confident in their role, and expertise, they should be able to establish easy rapport with the parents, who, after all, are the experts on their own offspring. This is quickly communicated to the parents and paves the way to truly integrated care. As parents become accepted as members of the team, it is easier to consider their needs with much the same care as is afforded the staff and patients. Their requests for meals, drinks, information, irritate staff no more than those of other members of the ward team. Even the consideration of admitting a sibling to facilitate a parent staying is part of the service.

Planning the Patient's Day

Much thought and adaptation may be required to make the patients' day, in a general district hospital, suitable to the needs of the young. The difficulties of doing this are magnified when the children are nursed alongside adults but can be successfully modified to accord with normal family behaviour.

MEAL TIMES

These can be made to coincide with those of the majority of homes. Few children are used to a cooked breakfast but most of them normally have their main meal at mid-day – but not before 12.30, which is the custom in some hospitals. Their preference for the evening meal seems to be fish fingers, sausages and chips, beans on toast. It has been my experience that once the catering staff understand the requirements, they are only too pleased to help. They are not always aware that children do not all delight in curries, liver, salads or the inevitable mince. Plated meal services are not very satisfactory for children and seem to produce a great deal of waste, especially when the whole meal is served together. It is unrealistic to expect children to eat their main meal before embarking on the more attractive dessert. This often means the protein, vitamins and roughage are left. When food is served from the old-fashioned trolley and mothers advise or assist, this is still the most acceptable method for the children's wards. Mealtimes are not a good time for most parents to go out, as they can be invaluable on most occasions to tempt their child to take nourishment. There are exceptions, of course, but if so, the staff will need to work with the parent to help establish better eating patterns.

Although 5.30 is late enough for the very young children,

the older ones will certainly welcome 'a little something' with a milk drink before going to bed. An interval of over 14 hours is too long between meals. Some children, unfortunately, are not used to regular meals and therefore some flexibility is required to meet their physical requirements. As many are not accustomed to eating breakfast at home, by mid-morning they may be ravenous. When the bigger children are well enough to roam, requests to visit the canteen or shop reveal a good trade in ham rolls from the paediatric departments. But if too many sweets are consumed before lunch, the taking of a well-balanced diet may become a problem. When children in the wards are on diets, it is particularly hard, especially as visitors tend to bring in all sorts of goodies, not all of which are nutritious!

MORNING ROUTINE

Fortunately most children seem to be able to sleep through tumult and take little notice of lights, once they have gone to sleep. Although some are exquisitely sensitive to noise and babies crying for example, others seem to sleep better amid a hubbub or interminable pop music. It seems to me quite unnecessary to wake them in the mornings, except for medication and I know of no good reason for them to be bathed, dressed and fed before the day staff arrive. It is alien to the average family routine and serves little purpose, providing the children are ready for school or play when the staff arrive. Sometimes children go out to school from the wards, others will need to be prepared for tests or operations. More time can be devoted to them if there is no mad scramble. At weekends, the timetable may be further relaxed. In one hospital I visited in Canada, the older children (in the adolescent ward) were allowed to sleep on in the mornings. They helped themselves to breakfast from a trolley left on the ward. This was one of the nicest things about the unit, they reported. And why not — is it so far-fetched?

BATHING

Traditions die hard and staff often feel they must bath all

the babies before the 10 am feed — despite the fact that parents cannot always get there in time and anyway there are usually more staff on duty after lunch. Similarly, nurses are reluctant to leave a child in the evening until Mummy or Daddy comes to bath and put him to bed. With very little re-organisation, this can be a real time-saver for over-pressed staff in the evening, and parents appreciate being allowed to do this for their child.

REST-HOUR AND BEDTIME

Some units preserve the hour after lunch for a rest-time. Curtains and blinds may be pulled to subdue activity. Others do not feel it is necessary for their patients. Whatever the policy, parents should never be given the idea they are not allowed to stay. It is often a good time for mothers to get a short rest, away from the demands of sitting at the bedside and sometimes they need encouragement to take the oppor-tunity. If the child is really restless without her, it may be important for her to be offered an alternative.

Bed-time may be a veritable 'movable feast', according to the age range of the patients. Whereas babies and most toddlers tend to be self-regulating when settled, as newly admitted patients they may be so disturbed as to be wakeful into the night and manage to keep everyone else awake too. To be able to pull down the blinds and dim the ward, rather difficult of course when the evenings are light, will help to settle the younger children. It also acts as a cue for the parents to tuck their children in and prepare to say good-night. The older children will become very bored unless permitted either to watch television, play quiet games or read for a while. It is usual for them to get to bed by the time the night staff arrive — unless they manage to persuade the staff that the programme is very suitable!

In our concern to provide a welcoming atmosphere it should be remembered that young children are traditionalists — they appreciate the security of a known routine. We need to provide a framework which will encourage our patients to feel secure and to 'know what happens next'. Routine has its place in a children's unit if only because of this. Discipline in the same way will enhance security providing it is fair, and seen to be fair, consistent and compassionate.

Summary

Providing a welcoming atmosphere excites the imagination. Looking at wards and departments from a child's point of view quickly shows easily remedied omissions. Even small adjustments to the patient's day can ensure children feel 'at home' with the routine. When children are only a small part of the hospital population, even small changes may involve patient negotiation. In some areas a radical change may be necessary. But adaptation of the traditional ward environment will mean these needs can be more adequately met.

Basic to the change, however, will be our own attitudes. How we express our love for the children, how we arrange nursing care and parental involvement so as to preserve that trust between child and mother. Discipline will become the loving, sensitive and consistent guideline that gives children security to know how far they can go. Encouragement will ensure each child, whatever his problems and handicaps, can achieve his potential with confidence.

References

British Paediatric Association (1974). *Planning Children's Departments,* London.

Oswin, M. (1971). *The Empty Hours,* Harmondsworth: Allen Lane.

Savage, John H. (1975). 'The Red Arrow', *The Nursing Times,* 20 November 1975.

Savage, John H. (1975). 'Anti-Climbing Hospital Cot Attachment', *The Nursing Mirror,* 17 May 1977.

Savage, John, H. (1977). 'Mattress Tilting Device', *The Nursing Mirror* 2 June 1977.

Shore, M.F. (1967). *Red is the Colour of Hurting: Planning for Children in a Hospital,* Washington DC: US Dept. of Health, Education and Welfare.

Organisation of the Patient's Day (1976). London: HMSO, Central Health Services Council.

Places Mentioned

Brook General Hospital, Woolwich.
Childrens Hospital, Vancouver, British Columbia.
Guys-Evelina Hospital, London.
Nottingham University Hospital.
Poole General Hospital, Dorset.
St Charles Hospital, Ladbroke Grove, London.

Part Three
The Ward Team

8 Management of a Children's Unit

Introduction

A great deal has been said about the needs of the sick child and his parents — how to make a hospital environment supportive and appropriate to them. The involvement of the ward team has been implicit, but nothing has been said about the very real needs the staff may have. Working on a children's unit is exacting. Nurses will need to combine a high degree of professional skill with patience and ingenuity as they care simultaneously for the varying needs of a wide age range. Their patients may be inconsolably unhappy, irrepressibly energetic, and impossible to keep in bed unless restrained in some way. Emotionally the staff may be acutely stressed by nursing a terminally ill child or because of a sudden death on the ward. Stress can be engendered too by anxiety of a parent or relative. Their repeated questions may react on staff who become defensive and hostile. The ward sister will have responsibilities to her students and pupil nurses who will need teaching as well as support in unfamiliar situations. Yet a happy ward is the reflection of a happy staff and a calm ward the result of confident, unified and sensitive management.

Children's wards can be the happiest wards in the hospital, with the most satisfied staff and patients. A nucleus of stable staff, good interpersonal relations and frank support in times of stress can be achieved.

Achieving Team Spirit

It is impossible to speak with one mind without knowing the whole story, having faced the problems and thought of the consequences. Traditionally wards have report sessions when the nurses are given details of condition, treatment and ongoing care of their patients. Rarely does this include emotional support. At times nurses are encouraged to talk about patients they have cared for that day. But it is not often that other members of the ward team are included. Obviously it is not possible for long involved comments to be given at the change of each shift. Night staff particularly tend to learn little about the 'other side' of their charges. One place I knew used to record on a cassette the main reporting session after lunch when there was time to talk about the family needs of the patients. This was then played over during the night when it was quiet. Many people feel internal rotation of staff can make continuity of care easier as there is more understanding of ward philosophy and the various agencies available to help.

WARD MEETINGS

Whether or not this is so there certainly needs to be a specific time when ward staff can get together to discuss problems, provide support and air new ideas. A change of nursing plan, the patients' day, the best time for ward rounds, meal-times, policy over relatives and friends, visiting later in the evenings, bed-times, rest hours — these matters need to be agreed so that junior members of staff know how to make decisions when they are 'in charge'. Flexibility does not mean lack of planning, a fact that seems forgotten in some wards.

It is always helpful if each discipline involved in the paediatric unit consults with the whole team before changing policy and these ward meetings make an ideal venue. In my experience the meetings need to be held every week and should include the learners as well as the professional members. Domestic staff who often have the easiest rapport with some patients and parents should not be forgotten. Although it can be a forum for learning about the medical or nursing care required by specific patients, problem-solving of behaviour, family difficulties and management of the ward can also be usefully discussed. In addition to those on the wards some hospitals run six-monthly open meetings to which *all* hospital personnel involved with provision of services for paediatric patients are invited. In this way, improved sensitivity to the particular needs of the young can be achieved right across the hospital service. It is encouraging that as child health services become more integrated, workers in the community are also being involved. It is always worthwhile spending time as an active participant of these meetings.

As well as the planned meetings, it has been my experience that informal conversations over a cup of coffee are invaluable in establishing mutual respect and cooperation. The rapport between doctors and nurses that results is so useful that I have always endeavoured to create such a haven where this can take place. It cannot be combined with a busy ward office, nor totally taken over by members of staff for their own professional use. It must be a multidisciplinary meeting place and involve the nurses; without them it loses much of its value. Yet in my experience they are the ones often most reluctant to participate.

MEETING CRISES

When a crisis has occurred on the unit it is very important to meet with the staff as soon as possible. For example, I was greeted one day by a nursing auxiliary who was upset 'They won't even have it christened. I think it's quite dreadful!' I soon discovered that a four-day-old baby had just been transferred to the unit from the local maternity hospital. He had an extensive meningomyocele involving neurological damage, and was to be given terminal care only. There was a great deal of unhappiness that the baby was not having a full complement of milk. The night staff had put down a naso-gastric tube as he was reluctant to take his feed. Because he was cyanosed, an oxygen cylinder was brought to the cubicle for use.

It was obvious that the whole issue needed to be discussed. What was the plan of care? Why was it that the child should not be made to take his full diet? What was the responsibility of the nurse? How could she provide all that instinctively she longed to do? Who was caring for the parents and particularly the mother? It transpired that the mother had requested that the baby be put in the incinerator after death! She had not seen the baby. Nor had anyone spent time talking with the parents about their feelings.

In tackling problems that touch such deep sensitivities in ourselves, it is quite obvious that time must be given, first to encourage each person to air feelings, and then to allow plenty of time to listen before giving guidance and support.

On another occasion, a seven-year-old girl about to be discharged inexplicably fell off her bed — dead. No amount of resuscitation had any effect. All that could be done was to waylay the parents (already on their way to collect her) and to break the news as kindly and gently as possible. There was no way that the other patients and parents could avoid knowing 'something had happened'. How much had they really seen? What should be the response if a child asked 'What has happened to Lucy?' It was urgent that the nursing staff should get together to discuss this. Did they feel the children should be told? Initially it was almost unanimous that the children should not. What would be the answer, then, if they asked what had happened? Removal to another ward? Gone home? It gradually became plain that none of the suggestions would be in any way adequate. Several then remembered what had happened when, as children, they had been told some untruth about the death of a relative or even an animal. It was finally agreed unanimously to tell all the children. The approach was made by asking each child and parent, where appropriate, if they had seen what had been going on. If so, what did they think had happened? In this way we were able to find out just how much had been witnessed. Most children asked outright if she was dead. One boy gave a graphic description of the resuscitation attempts. Asked how he had seen (we had been careful to screen the bed), he said it was reflected in the window behind. His reaction? He had wanted to get out of bed and help. So much for our ideas that children do not see! One adolescent, rather a vocal girl, and a bed patient on another ward on the lower floor, greeted me less than half-an-hour later with 'What happened to that child? She's dead, isn't she?' The grapevine is just as efficient in a children's unit.

There is value in regular get-together sessions between a member of staff and the parents. Successful meetings of this kind are held each week in certain hospitals for all parents, sometimes specifically for those whose children have similar problems. They may be organised by social workers, psychologists or ward sisters, although some units prefer not to involve ward staff as they are felt to inhibit free discussion.

Problems Specific to Paediatrics

There seem to be some problems that beset staff caring for children and their families. Where should one draw the line on untidyness? How many of the family does the child *need* to stay, and how can visiting siblings be cared for? It is to be hoped that insight into children's needs will make this sort of problem transitory and eminently solvable. Recognising there will always be problem parents, just as there are problem children, general policy should not change just because of their particular intrusions or violations of privilege. The stealing of equipment, for example, is a national problem. One famous hospital finally gave up furnishing a parents' day room because it had been stripped at least three times. Certainly hospitals I know regularly lose all the cutlery for the children and most of the special crockery too. Several times the electric kettle provided for the parents disappeared. The way to keep attractive items, I found, whether they were baby-bottle warmers, children's place mats, kettles, was to engrave them indelibly 'STOLEN FROM . . . . . . WARD'. It seemed that a souvenir with the ward name was not so desirable if it clearly indicated theft.

PARENTS

The ward team that supports and works together will be of most help to parents with problems, the member with the appropriate expertise and rapport taking responsibility. Where patient and, even better, *family* assignment is practised, it is much easier to establish continuity and it becomes more difficult for the problem family to manipulate the staff, an added advantage in an acute ward. When relatives come in their droves to visit, the sheer number may cause the most robust sister to quake. When the relatives make themselves at home, pick the best viewing chairs for the television, and take little or no notice of the patient they have come to see, one can understand that staff resent 'the invasion' and can see no good in the more liberal visiting arrangements. Children may find this behaviour quite normal and benefit from their presence more than those whose parents sit for hours at the bedside of their child, unoccupied and unnaturally attentive to every whim. To encourage a parent to busy herself and yet remain available, should her child need her, is ideal.

SIBLINGS

What about the other children of the family? If the hospital wants them to be with the sick child, it will be necessary for some parents to bring the rest of the family. Few hospitals have large enough children's wards to accommodate siblings all day. Fortunate units can provide 'lodging' for a sibling, when a parent wants to live in and find a spare cot or bed in the ward or in the mother's room. Of course, apart from feeding and bedding, the parent takes full responsibility. To feed visiting siblings is a difficult problem, especially where there is no visitors' canteen. Occasionally a sick child can be encouraged to eat if he sees his family doing so. Even with the strictest of rules, sometimes there seems an unusually large number of children at the table! There is also the problem of what to do to tempt the immigrant child or desperately ill patient to take nourishment at all. Parents may be only too willing to bring in some home-cooking. I well remember one child with a rhabdomyosarcoma who was desolate at not being able to go home and all she wanted was 'some of Mummy's Sunday lunch'. Ours just would not do. Mum was thrilled to provide some of course.

VISITING

Despite some of the headaches associated with open visiting, there will always be a few patients whose parents are elusive. There may be many reasons for this: a family tragedy; severe domestic stresses; parents who feel guilty about their child's handicap or threatened by the hospital; inability to afford travelling costs; anxiety about diagnosed abuse of their child (see Chapter 3) and, very rarely, abandonment. In all such instances the social worker and/or liaison health visitor should be alerted so that the best plans possible can be made with the community services. When a child is admitted following a road accident in which the parents are killed or injured, alternative plans are necessary. Other relatives may be recruited to fill the tragic gap. If not, the ward granny may provide a constant 'mother figure' (see Chapter 2).

Whatever feelings any of these situations evoke, the ward staff may need to take a positive supportive role towards the family. They must beware of the parent who feels my child 'will settle better if I don't visit'. Sadly this is a recurring comment made by some members of the public. 'My husband told me not to come as I only upset my child and myself'. Nurses can unconsciously reinforce this attitude when they say: 'Go home and don't worry — he'll be all right' and 'Oh, he was fine', when they phone to enquire. These families require encouragement and support from the nursing staff, to show them they are needed and wanted.

Because some children are admitted for well-defined physical causes, it may be unsuspected that there are deep family and emotional problems. It may only come to light when it is suddenly realised that no one has visited the child for some time. Unless it is a rule that visits are recorded, it may be impossible to give facts about the situation when asked. The task of social workers and health visitors will be much easier if entries include comments on parents' attitudes when with their child.

ACUTELY DISTURBED PATIENTS

Most staff on a paediatric ward breathe a sigh of relief when a specially destructive or hyperactive child is discharged. When the child suffers also from mental handicap, the problems may be even more acute. Staff in a busy children's ward are ill prepared to handle them. The decorations and amenities — quite safe and advantageous for a normally physically sick child — become hazardous and inappropriate for one attracted to the myriad of stimuli and yet unable to differentiate good from bad, what is allowed and what is not. Some of these patients, although at the inquisitive, touching, pre-school stage, may be chronologically and physically nearer adolescence. I have known one or two who have been irresistibly attracted to the tiny infants but who were totally unaware that they must not hit or throw them about. Others have been compulsive paper-eaters, with comics, toilet paper, tissues, all being found equally delectable. These children cannot be reasoned with for they do not comprehend that the resulting vomiting has anything to do with their unusual habits. Sedation can only be a mark of failure, but many units can do nothing else for the safety of the majority. It is sometimes very difficult to get such children transferred to the psychiatric division. They may indeed have come from a hospital for the mentally handicapped for assessment or treatment of physical disease; some are admitted regularly for dentistry under general anaesthetic. It can be an enormous relief if staff familiar to the children can accompany them. The sending hospital will sometimes allow the nurse to remain and 'special' the child and are always only too pleased to give advice and help in handling their patient.

Combined study days and liaison between the acute and specialist ward staff bring great reward. Not only is understanding of each other's problems improved, but so are skill and knowledge of specific paediatric conditions.

Health visitors and social workers also help to bridge the gap. Some of these children are being looked after at home by long-suffering parents and are admitted for respite care. In these instances the paediatric ward team may be able to give practical help which will alleviate the stress even after return home (see Chapter 9).

When suicidal boys and girls are admitted, the problems will be very different. The ward team approach is particularly important with this sort of patient. It may be that the child begins to develop a relationship with a junior nurse, auxiliary or play specialist. The rest of the team will do well to stay in the background, supporting her. Whoever she is, she will need guidance from the psychiatrist or specialist. Lines of communication must be good if those in charge are able to make accurate assessments and plan help. These children probably have difficulty in forming relationships with adults and their care will need great sensitivity and insight. The slightest ill-founded or unwise remark may have dire consequences. It may help the regain of confidence if he is well occupied and allowed to develop a meaningful relationship with a member of staff.

BARRIER NURSING AND CROSS-INFECTION

Nursing children in isolation requires the attention of all staff. It is more complicated when it involves parents, other visitors, and a large multidisciplinary staff. Yet unless it is simple, frankly, it will not be followed. Neither will it be implemented unless the necessary gowns, bags and so on are all at hand and in adequate supply. What nurse has not nearly cried in despair as she finds the doctor entering the cubicle oblivious to all instructions. Ward cleaners, too, may be sent from another ward 'to help' but trip happily from cubicle to cubicle without taking any apparent notice of the restrictions. Conversely, out of fear of infection, they refuse to clean at all and the cubicle becomes cluttered and dirty. Neither can it be assumed that nurses are blameless. Night and day staff do not always communicate well. Nurses come from adult wards because of staff shortages and may be unfamiliar with the precautions needed for children. Parents trying to be helpful may walk unconcernedly out of a cubicle holding an unprotected bed-pan.

There is no reason for the parents to be asked not to visit because of the danger of infection. They are quick to learn, provided the staff know exactly what they are doing and why. It may, though, be necessary to ask them to be extra careful in their own hygiene if they are living in. Children in isolation need their parents more, not less, as the barrier-nursing technique acts as a deterrent to more contact than strictly necessary by the staff. The wearing of masks needs to be rationalised and in many hospitals it is no longer policy. For the young patient's sake this cannot be anything but welcomed. When it is necessary it will help if the child can watch the nurse putting on her protective garments — and have a mask of her own to play with. When possible, the nurse caring for a child in isolation should be allowed more time to be with him. Isolation too often means a devastating separation and can be acutely lonely for the patient.

TRANSPLANTS

One of the newer problems to face paediatric staff is the potential child donor. Recently I was told of the first instance of this in one children's ward. The child in question had been admitted following a head injury. Nursed on a respirator for five days, it was decided the child was unlikely to survive. After several periods off the respirator and the usual tests, she was pronounced legally dead. The parents gave their permission for her kidneys to be used for a transplant. The child was prepared for theatre. Before being taken, the parents were advised to take leave of their daughter. They would not see her alive again. The staff felt this leave-taking acutely. The student nurses admitted to no conflicts. The trained staff who had nursed her were most upset. The difficulty seemed to be to accept the fact that the child must be kept breathing until the organs had been removed. In their minds they accepted life was only maintained by mechanical means. Emotionally they were quite unable to accept it was right. How could they help the parents through this sad time? For some parents the agony of watching a ventilated child may be so acute that there is a certain relief when a decision is finally made. This may be also true for staff.

Quite obviously this sort of problem cannot be handled by any one discipline. The medical staff play a crucial role in this, and one suspects that many never had the opportunity to experience the support of other members of the team. Yet it is their clinical expertise that will help the others rationalise their feelings about this sort of case. Some medical staff are able to admit to personal feelings and emotional conflicts, others not. Difficulties begin when, for whatever reason, true feelings are not expressed by any members of the team. On the surface it may be easier to blindly follow directives but the deep inner conflicts and hurts will manifest themselves. It may be shown by presenting a hard exterior — a brusque offhand manner that belies the true sensitivities of the individual.

Summary

In planning and staffing a paediatric unit, account must be taken of the very specialised skills and training required to meet the challenge of today's family-centred paediatrics. Not only will the staff need to be committed to these concepts, but they may have to develop new skills to cope with them. Because of integration with the child's home environment it is essential that staff have a working knowledge and understanding of the community services. It should be recognised that with these new concepts will come new and somewhat different stresses. Students and pupils must be strongly supported, as most of their work will be done in front of parents. Young doctors will probably need the same kind of support until they feel more confident in their techniques. Paramedical staff will want to feel fully integrated and valued members of the ward team. They should expect and receive the same support as the nurses and doctors. Staff can have the most satisfying job available to hospital personnel. More than gratitude of dependent patients, they can experience the exhilaration of working as a team with families in the fight against disease and handicap, and to see those families broken by a calamity begin to regain confidence to handle whatever hurdles remain.

References

Blake, F. (1954). *The Child, His Parents and the Nurse,* Philadelphia: Lippincott.

Central Health Service Council. (1976) *The Organisation of the Patient's Day.*

Committee on Child Health Services (1976). *Fit for the Future* (the Court Report), London: HMSO.

Hawthorn, P. (1974). *Nurse I want my Mummy,* Royal College of Nursing.

Hardgrove, R. and Dawson, R. (1972). *Parents and Children in Hospital,* Boston: Little, Brown & Co.

MacCarthy, D. and Morris, I. (1959). 'Mother and Child in Hospital — the Practical Aspects', *The Nursing Times* 55, 8, 219—222.

Menzies, E.P. (1961). 'Nurses Under Stress', *The Nursing Times*, 57, 5—7.

Oswin, M. (1971). *The Empty Hours,* Harmondsworth: Allen Lane.

Pillitteri, A. (1977). *Nursing Care of the Growing Family,* Boston: Little, Brown & Co.

Wolff, S. (1969). *Children under Stress,* Harmondsworth: Allen Lane.

9 Integration of the Ward Team

Introduction

Because good paediatrics concerns itself with the needs of the whole child, it is inevitable that it will draw on the expertise of many people. On the other hand Pamela Hawthorn in her Report *Nurse I want my Mummy* (R.C.N., 1974) warned that children both in general and specialist hospitals were suffering from 'this barrage of professionals'. Alongside our enthusiasm to provide a comprehensive service for children, the need for each member must be appraised carefully to ensure their contribution really is necessary.

Much has been said for unity in the ward team, the essential mutual respect that comes from a true appreciation of each other's role. Never is this more necessary than in the large multidisciplinary team involved in the children's unit. A short account will be given here of the unique role these rather specialised members play in a paediatric setting.

Liaison Health Visitor

In recent years, and particularly since the re-organisation of the health service, attempts have been made to bring together the community and the hospital services. Because of its preventive and community role, health visiting is ideally suited to bridge the gap. Health visitors are all general trained nurses, many of whom have other nursing qualifications. In addition they are required to have midwifery, or at least obstetric training. In the community they serve, they have responsibility for all children under five. In addition to this, some have a commitment to the family, including geriatric care. Their responsibility for children lies in infant feeding, developmental assessment in conjunction with community physicians and general advice on child-rearing, preventive medicine and immunisations, with special emphasis on family relationships and good health education.

The Court Report (1976) recommended that certain health visitors be given more responsibility for sick children in their own homes. In one or two areas, health visitors are being used in the care of acutely sick children, who otherwise might have been in hospital. Where this is so, it is imperative they have a recognised paediatric training and are in touch with current practice. When the health visitor is appointed to the ward she may be able to relay up-to-date paediatric practice back to the community, as some health visitors confess to a lack of this specialised knowledge. Her main task in the ward will be to keep her colleagues in the community informed of the young child in hospital; where necessary, to assist the parents and family during the admission, but certainly to ensure their follow-up after discharge. In some areas, she may also include any child seen in casualty, which can be particularly helpful when non-accidental injury is suspected. Her presence hopefully permits a potentially more comprehensive service. Health visitors are now taking an active interest in special-care baby units. Knowing the family circumstances enables some infants to be discharged earlier. The health visitor can give great assistance to the other members of the ward team when plans for on-going care are made. Her information on the locality may allow the true nature of the presenting problems to be more quickly recognised. In the forward-thinking areas she becomes a daily visitor to the ward, attends reports and doctors' rounds, as well as other unit meetings. Ideally, she should become a fully integrated member of the paediatric team. Unless she does, there is a likelihood she will not be used to her potential as her specialist knowledge brings a down-to-earth realistic approach to what is practical in the home environment.

Community Nurse

In a few areas, home-care schemes have been initiated with the express purpose of nursing sick children in their own homes, a direct alternative to hospitalisation. For some it means they do not go into hospital at all. Others may have had surgery or treatment as a day patient and then continue care at home (Southampton), whilst more chronically sick and handicapped children are able to benefit from a more normal life because it is not peppered with long boring visits to out-patient clinics. Schemes currently are running in areas as far apart as Southampton, London, Birmingham, Gateshead and Edinburgh. Each has a slightly different emphasis and is staffed according to available resources and willing commitment to the scheme. The majority are run from the community nursing services with members of their staff seconded to the hospital. At Southampton the doctor-in-charge admitted he almost forgot his 'Sister' wasn't actually on the staff of the hospital. They are all experienced well-qualified paediatric nurses. This is important when it is realised some of the schemes involve making clinical judgements and taking decisions on the condition of their patients. As children's health changes so rapidly, this can be a considerable responsibility. Some of their expertise will be needed to be utilised in teaching the parents, since the nurses will not be there continuously. There is an excellent home-care scheme in Montreal (see Appendix 1).

The staff in these schemes are unanimous in their enthusiasm, and report that patients and parents are equally appreciative. In view of the expense of hospital beds, and the known psychological damage that can occur as a result of separation, it is a sad reflection on the priority given to children in our country that home-care programmes have not become widespread.

Social Worker

The first social workers employed in hospitals towards the end of the last century were the 'almoners'. Today their role is very different and they are primarily concerned with the many social problems of patients and their families. Following the re-organisation of the health service in 1974, hospital-based social workers were assimilated into local authority social service departments. The big hospital centres still have a permanent social work staff based in them; in some places hospitals are serviced by social workers who come in from the community-based area teams.

Most paediatric units have a social worker and such a person is an integral part of the ward team. Broadly speaking her tasks are: to provide a direct case-work service to sick children and their families; to participate in medical and nursing teaching programmes; to alert the ward team to the implications of the social and emotional problems of their patients and relatives; to help support other members of the team with the many stresses they face in daily ward work. Since nurses work very closely to children and parents, where possible a daily dialogue with the social workers is to be encouraged. Nurses sometimes have 'hunches' about situations and family relationships which they may feel are not significant enough to report. Use the social worker to share these concerns. They may be important clues in understanding family situations.

Many problems can arise in family life as a result of illness or handicap and amongst ways the social worker can help are the following:

(i)   to facilitate parental visiting, which may include helping to make arrangements for the care of other relatives or pets, or even fund-raising to help meet travel costs.

(ii)   to act as a liaison person in coordinating aftercare for children who require help from statutory or voluntary sources, including the many self-help groups in the community.

(iii)   to be involved with children who may have been abused or who are at risk of being injured. In some areas this may include being involved in taking out a Place of Safety Order.

(iv)   to help parents around the crisis of diagnosis, especially when the doctor is having to give them bad news about their child. In some areas the social worker is alerted whenever a child is brought to the accident and emergency department, following a cot death.

(v)   to try to assess parental capacity to cope with the long-term problems of chronic disability and the numerous implications this can have in respect of the marital and family situation.

(vi) to ensure parents know what resources there are to help them with their child. For example: housing and house adaptations, nursery placements, residential care, entitlement to monetary allowances. They must also know how to reach such resources.

(vii) to help support parents emotionally whilst nursing their child in the terminal phase of illness. Important too is the help needed by healthy siblings for whom life may be severely disrupted. Parents experiencing such sadness and distress are sometimes unable to communicate with them and indeed be unaware of their needs, both materially and emotionally.

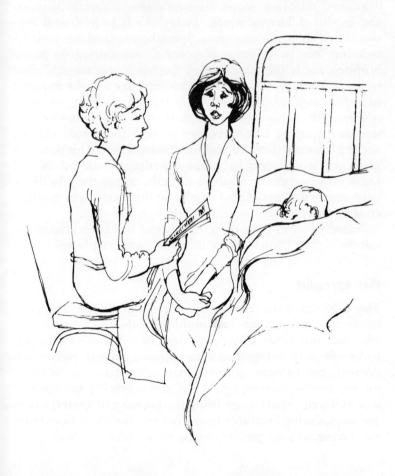

Within the ward, the social worker can help children to talk about their fears and feelings. This may reveal some of the underlying family tensions and alert the team to children who need further skilled help through the family psychiatric services. Children and parents are frequently referred through the out-patients clinics.

Nursery Nurse

Th nursery nurse is being used more and more in the health service, although she may no longer get any specific training in the care of sick children. Traditionally, she has been employed mainly in maternity wards, special-care baby units, and in the children's wards. Today she is to be found anywhere that children congregate. Special clinics and out-patients welcome her to organise play for those waiting. In many hospitals she is the 'play leader'. But her role remains blurred by her versatility. When the ward is busy she may be required to act as a nurse. Because she is trained she may be given responsibility for quite ill children. It is not always appreciated that her training has fitted her to care for the developing needs of normal healthy children under seven. This does not mean she will always have had experience with babies and know how to make up a baby's formula, one of the jobs likely to be assigned to her. Another may be the teaching of mothercraft to parents.

Nursery nurses have preferences, and when working in the sphere of their choice can be invaluable and irreplaceable.

Play Specialist

The play specialist has been created out of the unspoken needs of children who had nothing to do and nursing staff who had not time to occupy them. She has shown herself to be not only indispensable to harassed parents, nurses and doctors, but to have an increasingly important role in meeting the developmental, emotional and psychological needs of sick children. Apart from being the provider of games, paints and toys, she has been able to use her creative skills to enthuse the youngsters to participate in many activities and adopt play materials to meet a wide range of abilities and disabilities.

Normal development may be arrested during a traumatic experience such as being in hospital, but with the help of the play specialist he can be encouraged to resume his normal life-style. Working closely with other disciplines she can be the right hand of the nurse trying to perform a lengthy uncomfortable treatment. In similar ways, with the help of the play specialist, the physiotherapist, occupational therapist and speech therapist can often obtain ideas that will enlist the patient's cooperation with remedial treatment.

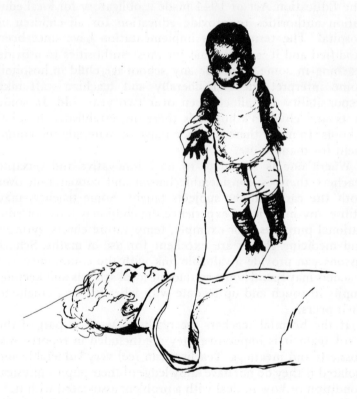

Another role that play specialists increasingly have is that of preparing children for the specific treatments or experiences they will encounter. This is somewhat controversial, as some feel it is the nurses' prerogative to prepare children for the care they themselves will be involved in (see Chapter 7). However this is perceived, it is essential that play and nursing staff work together in this very important field.

The main complaint about play specialists is that they are not available 24 hours a day, 7 days a week. No one could have a higher compliment paid them. They have certainly won their way into a permanent place in the ward team.

School Teacher

The Education Act of 1944 made it obligatory for local education authorities to provide education for all children in hospital. The terms of its implementation have since been modified and it is now usual for most authorities to provide teaching in some form for any school-age child in hospital. Some interpret the Act liberally and teaching staff take responsibility for all children over two years old. In some units and children's hospitals there are established hospital schools. In many there is a wide range of materials and equipment for them to use.

Where one is fortunate to have innovative and versatile teachers there is considerable liaison and cooperation over both the care and the subjects taught. Some teachers may utilise any material or experience the child may have for educational purposes. For example, temperature charts, syringes and medicine glasses are excellent for use in maths. School lessons can provide a valuable link with the community and teachers may spend hours contacting local schools and keeping pupils in touch and up to date with what is being taught to their peers.

If the hospital teachers are really to work as part of the ward team it is imperative they are included in reports, discussions and meetings. Teachers can feel very vulnerable and isolated if they do not have knowledge of their pupil's physical condition or how to deal with a problem associated with it.

Because of the erratic school population it is difficult for the teacher to plan ahead. She may also need to visit an older adolescent on an adult ward as well as care for the children's unit. Where she has no classroom to which children can come in a normal way, she will have to be content with bedside teaching, competing for her pupil's attention alongside the many distractions of an acute ward. Of course, these problems do not exist so much in a hospital catering for long-term conditions. Occasionally ex-patients may return in order to attend the hospital school as day patients.

Teachers, more than anyone else, provide a continuum of learning, part of normal living which may give the child patient the reassurance for which he craves.

Other Specialist Members

Mention should be made of some of the other members of the ward team even though they have significant roles with adult patients and may only visit children by request. These include dieticians, occupational therapists, physiotherapists, radiographers, speech therapists and technicians from the laboratories, ECG and EEG departments. Although working through parents may be unfamiliar to such personnel, where they combine expertise with empathy this enriches their contribution, indeed they may become very popular with their young charges and indispensable to their colleagues. Encouraging progress is being made today in the adaptation of highly complex equipment to meet the needs of child patients. One example of this is the new holding device used for securing babies who need to be X-rayed.

Chaplains and ministers of all faiths are not always familiar figures on the paediatric wards. Some years ago they were always called for if an infant was thought likely to die so that he could be baptised. This is no longer automatic. Thus parents and children may be deprived of the special solace and comfort those with a live faith can offer in times of stress. Where a chaplain has good rapport with children, he is a welcomed and popular figure who becomes an active member of the ward team.

This is equally true of the members of the psychiatric team when the hospital is fortunate enough to have them on the staff. At the Yale-New Haven Hospital the paediatric adolescent wards had daily visits from the consultant psychiatrist who was 'available in the unit' for any member of staff or patient. Sometimes I was told he just sat and had a cup of coffee, at other times was able to take the heat out of an emotional crisis engendered by some behavioural problem with a disturbed adolescent. The ward team relied heavily on his expertise and sensitive caring approach to staff and patients.

Summary

Paediatrics is concerned with the needs of the whole child. Thus it is not sufficient to provide expertise and personnel merely to meet the physical needs of children. Because of the many facets of care, there are an increasing number of specialists converging on the paediatric wards. Coupled with the shorter hours of duty and the rapid turnovers, both of staff and patients, it seems there are always new faces to be seen in the ward.

The permanent personnel on the ward provide a stable nucleus which is instrumental in creating a caring atmosphere. Thus ward hostesses, receptionists, secretaries and clerks need to share the ward philosophy and sense of commitment, just as much as the domestic and portering staff. It is the responsibility of the senior staff to ensure that they share this with them.

The mutual respect of each member of the ward team is enhanced when the unique contribution brought is fully recognised and utilised. Where it is possible to do so, the ward benefits if social workers and medical secretaries can be based within the unit. By fully integrating the ward team it is easier to rationalise the care any one family receives and cut down the number of different people to whom they are expected to relate. In this way not only do patients benefit but staff also have much greater job satisfaction.

References

Lightwood, R. *et al.* (1957). Home Care for Sick Children. *The Lancet,* 9 February 1957, 313–317.
Nash, S. (1976). *What is a Playworker?,* NAWCH newsletter, summer.

10 The Student in the Paediatric Ward

What's Special about Paediatrics?

The nursing of children can be totally demanding. It can be frustrating, stressful and exhausting, but it can also be fun. Powers of observation and sensitivity will be sharpened just because small children are so dependent on adults. Children find it difficult to tell you how they feel. They may not ask for what they need and their vocabulary may test your ingenuity – as well as burn your ears at times! But children are not isolated beings – they come in families.

This may be the basic reason why some students and pupils feel apprehensive. Confident of handling a patient, they may find the idea of including relatives in nursing care another matter. Do not worry about this. Relatives often feel far more nervous than you do. The whole of hospital is strange to them, not just the ward. If you show sensitivity to their feelings they will be 'on your side' and invaluable in helping in all sorts of ways to care for their child.

Children have specific growing needs which cannot be neglected, even while they are unwell. Nursing children therefore involves attention to their special needs which are often thought of as purely physical, but include emotional and social support from parents, staff and, for the older child, friends and relatives too. Play and education are also an important part of their daily life. It is partly because children are found in every part of a hospital — accident and emergency, out-patients, operating theatre, laboratories, X-ray, intensive care – that children's experience is mandatory in nurse training. The basic things to try to learn when seconded to the paediatric ward are:

to feel comfortable with children.
to see the needs of the whole child.
to communicate with them.

Learning to Feel at Home with Child Patients

Children's wards are designed to be less threatening and more like home than the rest of the hospital. Although it may seem chaotic at times, the atmosphere is intended to be deliberately informal and relaxed but you may still be facing issues of life and death in this unfamiliar set-up. Do take time to think out your own personal values before embarking on paediatrics. It is only in the children's and maternity wards that you are likely to face the clinical problems of treating or not treating congenitally handicapped or malformed babies. Death in a children's ward is an experience that often unexpectedly strikes deep emotional chords in human beings (see Chapter 8). But to be forewarned is to be forearmed. Make sure you can talk over these things with a friend — your tutor or your clergyman if you are in doubt.

Make yourself proficient at the normal tasks young patients will require and take the trouble too to learn how to hold a baby safely and firmly. Taking a baby's temperature, or even that of a young child, can be a hazardous business. There are wriggly babies and children who chew the end of a thermometer if it is put in their mouths. This is why there are rules about children of certain ages always having their temperature taken in the axilla or rectum.

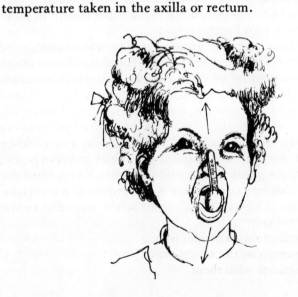

Giving medicines can be messy. Babies are not polite. They are adept at spitting out anything they do not fancy. Try putting the bowl of the spoon end on (not sideways) on to the tongue. Tip the handle up so it touches the nose and hold it there. It presses the tongue down slightly and, however much the infant objects, he cannot use his tongue to spit proficiently and the medicine goes down! The mother may be glad of this tip too. It is never really necessary to resort to holding the child's nose. You may have to wait for a howl before he will open his mouth but that's your opportunity. One of the reasons little ones have to come into hospital is to ensure adequate medication to control the infection, so it's good to know this tip. I have found it always works.

Feeding and toileting too can be made much easier if you handle the child with fairly firm confident movements – but talk to the child all the time. Make a game of any task whenever you can. Do not be afraid to use your imagination and remember children love games and stories repeated over and over again and do not forget that playing with a child is part of your role as a nurse. Mother and father can be included in the caring process almost always. Do get them to help you and show you 'how their child likes it done'. Having two of you, one to hold or divert the attention, is always good. The nurse who has the confidence to include the parent in whatever she is doing will find the procedure much easier. She will also learn a great deal from the way the parent does things. The intimate nature of the nurse's caring enables her to use her observations to help in the understanding and treatment of the child.

Recognising the Whole Needs of the Child

Although this has been dealt with in the earlier part of the book, as a student you will find it a great help if you observe how children of different ages react to the same situation — the sort of toys and games they play, what happens when they are tired, upset or hurt. Observe normal children on the bus, in the supermarket, out playing. Try to guess their age. Listen to their conversation. For example children get frustrated when they are not understood or cannot have what they want. Watch the two—three year old who wants an ice cream and is told 'No'. He is likely to scream, kick and even lie down in the street. Mother can often be seen dragging him along the pavement! The four—six year old may cry or whine. The older child will probably argue or wheedle in an attempt to get his own way.

Some schools of nursing arrange for their learners to spend time in the community before coming to the children's ward. Seeing how families in the locality live and how they deal with problems will make the nursing student more sensitive to family needs in the wards.

In recognising the needs of the child you will be expected to be alert to the child's physical condition. Do remember this can change with incredible rapidity. Deterioration in adults is much slower usually. With children you cannot afford to wait. Always report any change *at once*. As children rarely can tell you accurately about themselves, it is particularly important to look out for any signs or symptoms. Child abuse may be recognised as the result of an observant nurse reporting behaviour of a child that cowers or appears unexpectedly fearful. The appearance of bruising is most easily observed whilst bathing. Similarly the nurse may be the first person to notice projectile vomiting, rumination, *petit mal* or convulsions. It may be difficult to communicate with the child whose vocabulary is limited but, if the words used in the family for bowel action, urination, his bottle or special toy or blanket are recorded at the time of admission, this can be a great help.

Meeting the child's need to play, to hide, to play out his feelings about home as well as hospital will be part of this care. For example the very vastness of the ward can be intimidating and children seem to delight to hide away. Under beds, in 'tents' made of bedspreads, in corners. You will be popular if you offer a large empty cardboard box that they can actually crawl into. A working knowledge of the ages at which they are likely to respond in a given way and to need certain help will make it easier and more interesting to you as well as benefit your patients (discussed in Chapter 4).

Learning to Communicate

Children are fascinating individuals and often think and behave very differently from adults. By thinking of the impact of our words and how they can be interpreted, it becomes easier to get on their wavelength. Ask a little boy if he wants 'a bottle' or even a urinal. What does he think he is being offered . . . a bottle of lemonade perhaps? When the doctor requests a patella *hammer* and proceeds to use it, is it not certain to hurt? Using simple language to explain what you are doing, or want the child to do, will go a long way in establishing rapport.

Learning to communicate with children means that you will need to think hard how it felt when you were young. Children want to know what is going on. But they do not always understand adult vocabulary and certainly have strange interpretations of medical jargon. For example:

Robert, aged eight, had a fractured femur pinned some months before. He had returned to have the pin removed, now the leg had healed and grown. He remembered that his leg was to be made strong by the pin. But after surgery he could not be persuaded to get out of bed. He could not say why. Eventually we guessed perhaps he thought his leg wouldn't be strong enough without the pin. By looking at the X-rays together, he was finally convinced it was. He immediately got up and started running round the ward as normal.

Try listening to the children if you want to know how they are thinking. Give them time to tell you things. If they do not want to, then ask for example, 'What do you think that drip's for? Why have you got this hard plaster on your leg? How will they get it off?' You may be surprised to know how many quite old children think their own leg is no longer there. Remember to be simple, tell the truth and if you do not know the answer tell them so honestly. Children respect and ferret out the truth but they will not think less of you if you honestly do not know. I find it easy to say on these occasions 'Would you like me to find out?' Do so and then go back and tell the child at once.

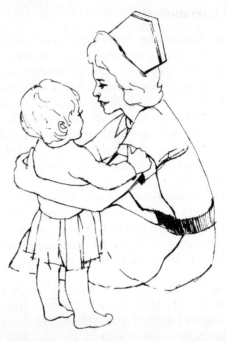

When talking to children, it is neither necessary nor kind to use 'baby talk'. But do try to talk at their level of understanding. Use simple everyday words and be prepared to repeat them over and over if necesssary. Speaking face to face, that is getting down to their height, either by sitting, squatting, or taking the child on your lap will mean there is less chance of your 'talking down' to them. Never be at a loss if your charge is homesick or cries. Cuddle him on your lap, carry him over your shoulder while you are working, but do not leave him to sob in his cot. And remember that the child who sits and stares, or rocks silently back and forth, may be even more unhappy. Little ones, that is babies and toddlers; the under threes, are a particular problem when they are in hospital without their mothers or fathers. It is not really possible to provide what they need — no one can adequately replace a parent and they cannot understand where Mummy or Daddy are. The ward granny, if she can stay 24 hours a day and devote herself as a normal mother would, to the sick youngster may be a substitute but failing this the nurse will find whatever she does is inadequate to the child's need. When a young child is homesick there is nothing for it but crying it out but cuddling by the nurse helps until sleep comes. Some units have small prams or push-chairs that are used in the wards. Children sometimes settle down if put in a familiar pram. This has the advantage too that the child can stay beside the nurse even when she is busy with other things (see p. 114).

When children are a little older it may be possible to divert their attention after a short cuddle and they may regain interest in some activity. This is not always so easy and the child may feel Mummy or Daddy will not come again. I have found that by 'phoning the parents in the presence of the child and sometimes with him on my lap so he can speak to them, he has been comforted by the familiar sound of their voices. He may cry at the time but afterwards seems more contented. This is more likely to be a help with children over four, whose understanding is greater. They can visualise time somewhat better so that the promise of the next visit can hold some meaning for him, especially if it is linked to a well-identified event such as a meal-time. Incidently it can show the parents that their presence is valued on the ward. Some parents still need encouragement to believe this.

If you have been asked to move a child's bed or cot, do not do this without preparing your young patient first. One little girl of four I thought I had prepared fully said she was happy to be given 'a room all of her own'. But as another nurse and myself wheeled her cot into the cubicle she sobbed inconsolably 'now Mummy not find me'. What she needed was reassurance on this. We should have waited until Mother was there. This sort of anxiety seems quite common with children of all ages, but one that mystifies adults, who would expect a parent to ask where the child was. If children appear reluctant to move or go to the playroom for example, it can be a good idea to write a big note with the child, 'Mummy, Johnnie has moved to' or 'Mummy, I have gone to the play-room', which can then be left in a prominent position on the child's pillow or locker. By being sensitive in this way, you will be doing more for your patient than you may realise.

When you admit a child, do be truthful. One little boy of

seven, on learning in the evening that he was not going home as his mother had promised, but had come into hospital for a minor operation, told me 'I'll never trust my mother again.' What a tragedy and so unnecessary. If we had taken time to support the mother in the beginning, she could have been helped to face her child with the truth. A nurse is often heard to tell a mother to 'Go home and have a good rest.' How can a mother whose child is sick, really rest? If her child was crying when she left, guilt and fear for her child 'left' in hospital may be all the greater. We need to be more aware of the effects of what we say.

One of the main complaints of parents living in with their children is that they are not woken in the night even when the child has an injection or treatment. The night staff feel they can handle the child as he is likely to go back to sleep without disturbing the parent who 'needs the rest'. Parents quite rightly point out that this is the very reason they have elected to stay in. Should their child wake, they really *want* to be called, however tired they may be. Those whose domestic responsibilities make it impossible to stay like to feel that if they wake up in the night at home they can find out by telephone just how their 'baby' is. To hear 'Hang on a moment, I'll go and have a look', followed by a truthful report, even if it is to say he is upset, can be strangely reassuring to an anxious mother. You can be sure that if you say 'He's slept all night' with the idea this is kinder, some other parent will relay the truth and the result will be that the parent will be more anxious, not less.

The Challenge

To find yourself constantly in the shop window, to be always 'on show' to the parents and relatives may be a shock. If you just remember that whereas you are anxious lest the parents criticise your efforts, they will be equally anxious lest you think they are bad parents. You may feel unsure that you can gain the child's cooperation and will be ham-fisted over whatever you have to do. They will regard any 'playing up' by their child as evidence that *you* think they cannot control their own child. His crying may be the result of your hurting him – it may equally be the pain of bewilderment and fear. Spending a little time getting to know the parents will give the child a chance to learn that you are his parents' friend and therefore he can trust you. It will also help to relieve the parents, so they will be better able to cooperate with you.

Sometimes parents are so anxious to appear grateful for what is being done for their child that they fail to recognise his misery. But never ignore anyone who complains their child is not so well. Always report this *at once*. Parents are much more in tune with their own child. Every good paediatrician will tell you that if a mother says there is something wrong, you should believe her — even if there are no signs or symptoms. Parents will be your best ally. They are willing helpers and if you are willing to learn, can give you wise and practical help. But never just 'leave them to it' as they will need your support even if they do all the 'doing'.

If you are left in charge of a child or group of children, you may worry as to whether they will do as you tell them. When nursing children the cardinal rule is to be consistent. Do not say something unless you mean to carry it out. Even with small things such as taking medicine never ask a child 'Will you take this for me?' unless you are prepared for him to answer 'No'. If there is no choice, do not imply that there is one. The same applies to matters of discipline. It is no good saying 'Bobby you must stay on your bed' if you give in later. It can, of course, work two ways. I remember very clearly one night I was giving the night report when one four year old was still awake. She had been in a real pickle during the evening and had been out to the toilet on several occasions. 'Can I go to the toilet?' she interrupted during the report. 'No Jill you can't.' 'But I want to go', she replied in urgent tones. 'I'm sorry Jill, but you have already been twice. You must stay in bed.' Within a couple of minutes Jill stood up on her bed and began to micturate. I have never heard such a torrent. Her bladder must have been bursting. None of us dared turn round, nor could we show our mixture of mirth and annoyance. Fortunately we did not have to wash the bed linen!

Painful procedures, even the giving of injections, can evoke anxiety in the nurse just as much as in the young patient.

Never try to do anything on your own which you find difficult. Always enlist the help of either a parent or another nurse. Never approach a child suddenly or without warning — but neither give so much warning that you create more anxiety. I once saw a nurse 'preparing a patient' to have a naso-gastric tube passed. Every half-hour during the morning she went up to say "You do know . . . don't you?' You will be unlikely to be asked to undertake any complex procedure on a child without the assistance of a well-experienced paediatric nurse. Listen to the way she explains what is to be done, although it is unnecessary and unwise to give details. What is important is to truthfully answer any questions. For example, I might talk about using a very soft bendy straw to get rid of any 'sickness' but would not mention putting it down the nose — unless asked. Obviously, whilst actually doing the procedure, this would have to be explained — but not before.

The Rewards and Summary

There is a positive side to nursing children. They will demand the utmost from you. They will challenge your skills of observation, and remind you that their whole future may be in your hands. By their very vulnerability, physically and emotionally, they will expect your love and gentleness to comfort and console them, however naughty they may be. Without your sensitive and consistent caring they will feel insecure and isolated. Play with them, talk with them and, above all, listen to them — you will be amazed at their imagination and individuality and you will love them.

Dr Barry Brazelton from Boston, USA, has some encouraging words to say about children who have come into hospital. He believes even young school children can learn some very positive things from being in hospital, 'even from an operation, if it is properly handled'. He says a child learns a great deal from stressful situations, about himself and his ability to manage. Even though doctors and nurses hurt him sometimes, he learns they want to help him and he gathers confidence in himself and in other people. All this can be a positive experience in learning to master the world. Providing, of course, he gets the right kind of help.

What a child learns in hospital is to a great degree dependent on us. If we are sensitive and honest in our approach, anticipate and meet the total needs of the whole child, bearing in mind his age and developmental needs, then we can be confident he has a chance to emerge from this devastating experience a richer and more mature person. If we are committed to including the family in the care of each sick child, then the family, too, can emerge stronger and more united to face stress in the future. Child and family will have remained intact throughout what may have been the most difficult time in their lives.

Our part is crucial. Nursing children will demand more than we may have anticipated. But there can be no greater reward than seeing a child safely restored to health within his own family setting, knowing it was possible to protect him from many of the negative emotional experiences associated with hospitalisation and separation.

References

Barton, P.H. (1962). 'Play as a Tool of Nursing', *Nursing Outlook*, 10, 162.

Bergman, A.B., Shrand, H. and Oppé, T. (1965). 'A Paediatric Home-Care Programme in London: 10 Years' Experience', *Paediatrics*, 36, 314–321.

Blake, F. (1954). *The Child, His Parents and the Nurse*, Philadelphia: Lippincott.

Brazelton, T.B. (1969). *Infants and Mothers: Differences in Development*, Dell Publishing Co.

Homan, W. (1969). *Child Sense*, Basic Books, New York.

Homan, W. (1970). *Child Sense*, London: Thomas Nelson.

Leach, P. (1977). *Baby and Child*, London: Michael Joseph.

11 The Way Forward

Once we are convinced that young children should not be separated from their parents and that all children have 'growing needs' that require attention, we shall find ourselves establishing new priorities for their care in the wards of our hospitals. Once these priorities are accepted, it is merely a matter of working through the 'details' with imagination and sensitivity.

None of us can be satisfied, though, until there is not a single persistently unhappy, homesick and uncomforted child to be found in hospital. Whilst one bewildered and uninformed parent is allowed to remain this way, whilst the training of any future doctor or nurse lacks adequate teaching of the developmental and emotional needs of children, whilst staff of any discipline find it difficult to communicate meaningfully with their young patients, no paediatric member of staff dare assume she is providing the care she should to meet the total needs of the child.

Traditionally, specialised medical and nursing care has been provided within hospitals. Although this no longer means children are separated absolutely from their parents, we should already be going further — looking for even better alternatives. It may be possible to provide 'good enough care' to keep them out of hospital altogether. Our concepts of the nursing role may undergo further change. Adaptations and alternatives may need to be sought to protect the vulnerable 'under threes' who need specialist hospital care.

Certainly it is my conviction that we have only just begun to act on the implications of present knowledge. We all have much still to learn and even more to put into practice. Meanwhile the rewards of imaginative and innovative programmes are great and, more important, our children stand to benefit from them. The future indeed is an exciting prospect.

Appendix 1:
Alternatives to Hospitalisation

Home-Care Schemes

In some areas home care for the acutely sick child is practised. At present, most of the schemes are innovative and experimental, are run entirely by nurses and are linked with the community nursing services (see Chapter 9). In Southampton and London (St Mary's, Paddington) for example, the staff are seconded to the hospital paediatric team. In Birmingham, Edinburgh and Gateshead, it is part of the community service. One of the best home-care schemes I have seen was centred in the Children's Hospital, Montreal, Quebec, Canada. This was staffed with hospital personnel, had a 24-hour, 7-days-a-week medical and nursing service available to acute and chronically sick patients living within a 50-mile radius. In addition to the paediatrician and three nursing sisters, there was a social worker and physiotherapist on the team, with the services of a dietician and psychiatrist available. Children were not only discharged much earlier from the wards but many were sent home direct from casualty. Patients I saw included a 16-year-old boy on a respirator, a three-year-old with an acute infection superimposed on Wernig Hoffman's disease, a child with rheumatoid arthritis, a haemophiliac and chronic asthmatics.

When such a scheme was contemplated in a London suburb, it was calculated that at least 30 per cent of medical in-patients would benefit directly from such a service. If it included surgical patients, as is done in Southampton, where this is the main use of the scheme, it was anticipated that many more would be able to be cared for in their own homes. Even without special schemes there are an increasing number of children being discharged early with the cooperation of the community nurses. In one unit I know, the under threes with fractured femurs and — to an extent — those on abduction traction for congenital dislocation of hip, are sent home on traction, either with mobile apparatus or occasionally complete with hospital cot.

Self-Help Hospital Programmes

There are several hospitals in Canada and the United States I have visited who have pioneered what is known as 'Care by Parent Units'. Here, either in motel-type, purpose-built accommodation or an adapted ward complex, each family was allocated a room where the patient and parents stayed. In some instances a sibling was admitted too. There were communal dining and lounge facilities, kitchen and washing areas. More importantly each room had a telephone so that help could be summoned immediately if required. Doctors, nurses, as well as paramedical staff, visited but did not necessarily remain on the unit. Parents were taught how to take tests, provide treatment, give all their own drugs and take responsibility for the 24-hour supervision of their child. Such units were not suitable for all conditions but experience showed that the main criteria for admission was not so much degree of sickness, but the parents' ability and willingness to take the responsibility. Although the economic advantages of such units may play a part in their popularity in the United States, this was not the case in Vancouver. Yet this unit was equally well supported. The value of this type of care to the child and parent should not be dismissed.

Day Care

Many hospitals in this country have day-care units. Some are associated with the accident and emergency departments, others within the paediatric wards, and some have purpose-designed separate accommodation. Mostly initiated for minor surgery, paediatricians are beginning to use the same sort of scheme for children needing medical investigations. The disruption of the child's life is somewhat mitigated as he is able to go home at night. With instructions, most parents are willing and able to attend to the collection of any specimens or observations that may be required.

Appendix 2:
Questionnaire for Parents before Diabetic Children are Discharged

1. What part of the body is at fault in diabetes?
2. What are the common symptoms of uncontrolled diabetes?
3. How is diabetes controlled?
4. How can you test urine for sugar? Describe how to do it.
5. (a) When should you test urine?
   (b) How often?
   (c) What should you be careful of?
6. How is insulin given to a diabetic?
7. Which insulin acts quickly?
   Which insulin takes a long time?
   Which lasts longer?
8. When should insulin be given?
9. How do you keep syringes clean?
10. How many times can you use each needle?
11. What causes lumps in the places where injections are given?
12. If you break the needle when giving the insulin, what should you do?
13. (a) What is hypoglycaemia, or a 'hypo' attack?
    (b) What causes this?
    (c) How can it be prevented?
14. What are the symptoms of hypoglycaemia?
15. How should you treat hypoglycaemia?
16. Does the insulin need to be adjusted the next day?
17. If extra exercise is taken, how do you prevent a hypoglycaemic attack?

18. Which insulin affects the urine tests?
     (a) At noon?
     (b) Before breakfast?
     (c) Before supper?
19. Is it wise to change your insulin dosage frequently?
     Why?
20. Which tests of the day can show sugar without there
     being need for concern?
21. Would you worry if all tests of the day were blue?
     What would you do about it?
     (a) That day?
     (b) The following day?
22. What are the causes of diabetic coma?
23. What are the symptoms of diabetic coma?
24. How will urine tests show during an approaching coma?
25. Give rules for prevention of diabetic coma.
26. What should you do during illness?
     (a) With vomiting:
     (b) Without vomiting:
27. What foods contain mainly:
     (a) Carbohydrates:
     (b) Protein:
     (c) Fat:
28. What foods have little or no food value?
29. How many meals per day should a diabetic have?
30. Are there any special precautions you need to take?
31. If you found a stranger unconscious on the street and
     wearing a card or bracelet stating that he was a diabetic,
     what would you do?
32. Can a diabetic child grow up to be a heathy adult cap-
     able of marrying and having children?
33. How can a diabetic child reach that goal?

'Old' Diabetics

What is the most difficult part of managing your diabetes for
you?